American Melancholy

Critical Issues in Health and Medicine

Edited by Rima D. Apple, University of Wisconsin–Madison,
and Janet Golden, Rutgers University, Camden

Growing criticism of the U.S. healthcare system is coming from consumers, politicians, the media, activists, and healthcare professionals. Critical Issues in Health and Medicine is a collection of books that explores these contemporary dilemmas from a variety of perspectives, among them political, legal, historical, sociological, and comparative, and with attention to crucial dimensions such as race, gender, ethnicity, sexuality, and culture.

For a list of titles in the series, see the last page of the book.

American Melancholy

Constructions of Depression in the Twentieth Century

Laura D. Hirshbein

Rutgers University Press

New Brunswick, New Jersey, and London

Library of Congress Cataloging-in-Publication Data

Hirshbein, Laura D., 1967–

  American melancholy : constructions of depression in the twentieth century /
Laura D. Hirshbein.

    p. ; cm.—(Critical issues in health and medicine)

    Includes bibliographical references and index.

    ISBN 978–0-8135–4584–4 (hardcover : alk. paper)

    1. Depression, Mental—History—20th century. 2. Depression, Mental—United States
History—20th century. I. Title. II. Series.

    [DNLM: 1. Depressive Disorder—history—United States. 2. History, 20th Century—United
States. 3. Psychiatry—history—United States. WM 11 AA1 H663a 2009]

    RC537.H563 2009

    362.196'8527—dc22

                                             2008048083

A British Cataloging-in-Publication record for this book is available from the British Library.

Visit our Web site: http://rutgerspress.rutgers.edu

Manufactured in the United States of America

Typesetting: BookType

To Abigail and Daniel

Contents

Acknowledgments   ix

Introduction   1

Chapter 1   Prelude to Depression   9

Chapter 2   The Expanding Diagnosis of Depression   27

Chapter 3   American Moods and the Consumer Solution   57

Chapter 4   Gender, Depression, Diagnosis, and Power   77

Chapter 5   Feelings and Relationships   107

Epilogue: Real Men, Real Depression   127

Notes   135

Index   191

Acknowledgments

This project was supported by a publication grant from the National Library of Medicine and a grant from the Rachel Upjohn Clinical Scholars Program at the University of Michigan.

A precursor to this book was presented at the 2003 annual meeting of the American Association for the History of Medicine. I want to thank the numerous individuals who made helpful constructive comments, as well as the anonymous reviewers who provided assistance with the published version of that talk ("Science, Gender, and the Emergence of Depression in American Psychiatry, 1952–1980," *Journal of the History of Medicine and Allied Sciences* 61 [2006]: 187–216). I also want to thank Jennifer Gunn and John Eyler, whose gracious invitation to speak at the University of Minnesota in 2007 helped me polish the sections of the book on gender and depression.

As a clinician and historian, I am fortunate to be able to move in two communities, both of which have been encouraging as I have worked on this book. I want to thank the students, residents, nurses, social workers, activity therapists, administrative staff, and my faculty colleagues on both the inpatient unit (9C) and psychiatric emergency room (PES) at the University of Michigan Hospital. The teamwork has been inspiring, and my conversations with numerous individuals in these settings have helped to shape my historical arguments about depression. I also want to thank the faculty leaders in the department, especially Oliver Cameron, Gregory Dalack, Rachel Glick, John Greden, David Knesper, Michelle Riba, and Elizabeth Young, who have supported me in this incredible job in which I get to take care of patients and write history.

The community of historians of medicine has been wonderful as a source of both inspiration and support. Thank-you to Mary Fissell, Joel Howell, Margaret Humphreys, Howard Markel, Alexandra Stern, and Daniel Todes, all of whom provided important guidance. I also want to particularly thank the history of psychiatry community, especially John Burnham, Ellen Dwyer, Benjamin Harris, Jonathan Sadowsky, and Nancy Tomes, for their help with navigating the process from an idea to a manuscript. Thank you especially to Mark Micale for his support, his critical comments, and his encouragement to ask challenging questions. My biggest thank-you goes to Gerald Grob. Gerry has not only been a constant source of inspiration with his own outstanding work, but also he has helped me through conversations, with advice, and by reading my manuscript at a critical juncture. I feel honored to have had the opportunities to learn from him and to enjoy his company.

The process of turning the manuscript into a book has been a positive learning experience thanks to the Rutgers University Press, especially series editors Janet Golden and Rima Apple. I also owe a huge thank-you to Doreen Valentine, who not only edited the manuscript but also challenged me to better articulate my thoughts.

Finally, I want to thank my closest communities in Ann Arbor. I cannot possibly list everyone who has wished me well in this endeavor, supported me through the rough spots, or celebrated with me as I finished. I do need to thank especially Alison Davidow and Jim Rowe, Bob Davidow and Susan Grubb, Jessica and Omus Hirshbein, and, most important, Peretz, Abigail, and Daniel Hirshbein. Thank you all so much, and I hope I can be there for you as much as you have been there for me.

American Melancholy

Introduction

If you read about depression anywhere today—medical journal, popular magazine, National Institute of Mental Health (NIMH) pamphlet, or pharmaceutical company drug promotional literature—you will find three main pieces of information either explicitly stated or strongly implied: depression is a disease (like any other physical disease), it is extraordinarily prevalent in the world, and it occurs about twice as frequently in women as in men. The usual evidence marshaled to support these assertions includes clinical trials of patients responding to medications, World Health Organization statistics on the global burden of depression, and epidemiological data on the sex ratios in depression. All of this information sounds very compelling and scientific.

Perusers of popular magazines a century ago would not have been able to find depression mentioned as a disease, or even as a state of mind. The concept of depression in the popular realm referred to an economic, not an emotional, condition. Yet now depression is everywhere. Magazine readers will find frequent mention of depression in their favorite periodicals, from *Newsweek* to *Ladies' Home Journal* to *Sports Illustrated* to *Parents Magazine*. Popular accounts typically include the specific symptoms of depression, some explanation about treatment, and often patient stories of their experiences with depression. Commentators from public policy experts to physicians to journalists to patients discuss the tremendous extent of depression and its cost to society in time, resources, and human suffering. All of these accounts include the basic scientifically sounding facts of depression's status as a disease, its prevalence, and its predominance in women.

It would be tempting to see the emergence and proliferation of information about depression over the last century as evidence of scientific progress and discovery. Yet on closer inspection there is clearly more to the story, particularly around the issue of depression and gender. When I was in medical school and heard about depression the first time, I was immediately struck by the assertion that it was twice as common in women as in men. I started to look into this and ask around, but I was deeply unsatisfied by the answers I received from both my senior supervisors and the literature I consulted. In essence, the explanations given were: there is something in women's brains (probably related to estrogen) that produces depression; women's response to stress is to make them depressed; and, most commonly, depression has occurred more in women throughout recorded history.

I have to confess that I was suspicious of the claim that depression had *always* been more prevalent in women. (I had learned enough by that point in my training to know that the claim to eternal tradition was usually attached to a deeply ideologically driven practice.) As to the other two possibilities, I wondered about the men who were diagnosed with depression (what was wrong with their brains—too much estrogen?) or who were experiencing the same stress as women but were not apparently getting depressed. What about the other major lopsided mental illness statistic—that men suffered from substance abuse disorders at least twice as often as women? Was there a connection? The supposed sex difference in depression was also troubling because the diagnosis seemed somewhat arbitrarily defined (five out of a possible nine diagnostic criteria) and strongly suggested gender and power differences rather than simple biological sex differences.

As I looked into the history of depression, I discovered that it was *not* well established that women had always suffered from depression more than men. In fact, there was no specific disease of depression prior to the 1980 edition of the American Psychiatric Association's *Diagnostic and Statistical Manual-III* (*DSM-III*)—although there were disease categories of manic-depressive psychosis and involutional melancholia that shared a few of the same features as the current diagnosis of depression. Further, I discovered that the vast majority of clinical trials of medication for depression from the 1950s through the 1990s were done on predominantly female populations of patients, even before patients were selected for trials based on diagnosis or symptoms.

As I pursued my inquiry about gender and depression, I was more and more struck by how much depression has become almost exclusively perceived as a woman's disease in both medical and popular settings. In 1995, a *Time* magazine cover story on depression showed a picture of a solitary woman looking down at a coffee cup—the picture (which was actually a reproduction of Edward Hopper's 1927 painting *Automat*) seemed to imply that any woman who was alone without a smile on her face might be suspected of being depressed. In 2006, I had the opportunity to participate in a continuing medical education program about twenty years of progress in depression and its treatments. Several of us wanted to illustrate the program with a shadowy figure—the darkness of the photo suggested depression without necessarily committing to the sex of the potential victim. The education office instead chose a close-up photo of a young woman with glasses, staring down at something while holding her head. These, then, are our pictures of depression.

What is depression? The current diagnostic nomenclature of the American Psychiatric Association (APA), the *DSM-IV-TR*, states that the symptoms of depression consist of five or more of the following over the same two-week period: depressed mood most of the time, decreased interest or pleasure, significant weight loss or gain or appetite change, insomnia or increased sleep, psychomotor agitation or retardation, fatigue or loss of energy, feelings of worthlessness or excessive guilt, decreased ability to think or concentrate, and recurrent thoughts of death and/or suicide. The diagnosis is supposed to specifically exclude other things that could produce these symptoms, including drug or medication effects, general medical problems, or bereavement (unless the symptoms last longer than two months after the loss, at which point they would be considered symptoms of depression).[1]

The primary treatment for depression recommended by most psychiatrists is medication. There are a number of medications on the market, from older generic drugs to newer, expensive, and heavily marketed brands. Depending on insurance and patients' interests, patients might be referred for some form of psychotherapy.[2] While there are some who participate in longer-term psychoanalytic or psychodynamic treatments—forms of therapy that focus on the relationship between the patient and the therapist and how that relationship enacts older, more significant relationships for the patient—most of the patients who engage in psychotherapy today work on shorter-term treatments. Some of these forms of therapy are unstructured and are mostly supportive. Others are highly structured and involve homework, worksheets, and specific tasks to be accomplished within the therapy.

Over the last two decades, there have been significant efforts by a variety of individuals to educate the public and the nonpsychiatrist portion of the medical profession about the prevalence of depression. These campaigns have been local as well as national, and have involved efforts by psychiatrists, NIMH researchers, and pharmaceutical companies. At the same time that people across America have been educated to monitor their blood pressure, cholesterol, and potential for diabetes, Americans have also been warned to look out for the signs and symptoms of depression.[3] The campaigns about depression have generally been quite optimistic in tone, and have stressed that most people get better with either medication or therapy or a combination of the two.[4]

The significant increase in national attention toward depression over the last several decades has not passed without controversy, however, much of it centered around the role of pharmaceutical companies in marketing their products. In 2003 and 2004, reports began to circulate that selective serotonin reuptake inhibitors (SSRIs), a major class of antidepressants that includes agents such as fluoxetine (Prozac), paroxetine (Paxil), and sertraline (Zoloft), significantly increased the risk for suicide in children and adolescents. Not only was the risk alarming in and of itself, but also it raised questions about how the Food and Drug Administration (FDA) was helping to assure safety for psychiatric medication prescription since the majority of psychiatric drugs had not been tested in children.[5] By 2008, the controversy had not yet ended—the FDA required a black-box warning on antidepressants that indicated the possible risk, but this warning was denounced by psychiatrists as increasing the risk of suicide from untreated depression. Since suicide is a relatively rare event (compared to the large numbers of children and adults treated for depression), it is difficult to evaluate these claims one way or another. Still this controversy added to concerns voiced by many that diagnosing and treating individuals for mental disease was not necessarily a risk-free enterprise.

The business of psychiatric medication prescription has also received a fair amount of public attention, and psychiatrists have been under increasing pressure to disclose their financial and business ties to pharmaceutical industries.[6] Critics inside and outside the profession have pointed out the extent to which psychiatrists are shaped by their assumptions about medications, and how perniciously influential the pharmaceutical industry has become.[7] Yet as tempting as it is to externalize the problem—to view the pharmaceutical industry as the megavillain in a John Grisham–type novel—the story of psychiatrists' prescribing and diagnostic patterns is not solely driven by pharmaceutical company interest. As we will see in the case of depression, psychiatrists have had their own compelling professional reasons to promote depression as an illness.

Why are we ready and willing to believe the extraordinary prevalence rates of depression in our population? Can something that common really be a disease? Investigators who have studied other phenomena have certainly reached different conclusions about the relationship between prevalence and disease definition. In the early 1960s, Alfred Kinsey surveyed a large population of men regarding their sexual practices and found that approximately 10 percent of men engaged in exclusively homosexual relationships. In a thinking process that is striking in hindsight, Kinsey concluded that anything done by 10 percent of the population could not be considered evidence of diseased behavior and must in fact represent normal variation. Kinsey's conclusions about the normality of homosexual behavior helped to eliminate homosexuality from a list of diseases in the APA's *DSM-II* in 1973.[8]

Psychiatric epidemiologists and psychiatrists have not used the same reasoning as Kinsey, however, with regard to the normality or abnormality of very common patterns of behavior or experiences. Without any apparent second-guessing or questioning of the data, researchers have investigated what now constitute symptoms of mental illness and have claimed that 30 to 40 percent (or more) of the American population has or will suffer from a mental illness sometime in their lives. Are we really that diseased as a society? Or, as some critics have argued, have we expanded the definition of mental disease to the point of absurdity?[9]

In 2004, market analysts estimated that the sales from the global prescription of brand-name antidepressants totaled $14 billion—$9.9 billion in the United States alone. As pharmaceutical companies are well aware, the diagnosis of depression—and, more important, its treatment—represents very big business.[10] Depression research is also big business in a different sense for psychiatrists who have invested time, effort, and grants in developing an ever-expanding definition of depression. Further, millions of Americans seek out professional help for a variety of symptoms, including vague low feelings, difficulties enjoying their lives, and suboptimal social or occupational functioning. For these individuals, depression represents an important entity that will provide a name and a treatment for their experiences. Apart from a series of scholars lamenting the astronomical increases in psychiatric influence and diagnostic categories, there are few stakeholders advocating for the process of *reducing* national emphasis on depression.[11]

Where did all the energy and enthusiasm for depression come from? Where did it start, and what gave it such momentum? This book explores the history behind the rise in depression as a disease category with a focus on the twentieth century, the time period that has witnessed most of the important changes that explain the current focus on depression. Depression, like other diseases, has been constructed by social, professional, cultural, and gender forces around it. While the construction of disease in general has been a fruitful topic for many historians, psychiatric illnesses are particularly interesting to study because so much of what we think of as mental illness has changed over time within transformations in American society and the medical specialty of psychiatry.[12] The history of depression illustrates important shifts in physician practice and theory, professional issues within medicine, cultural factors regarding mental health and illness, and the gender basis of mental health. While science has been an important factor in the evolution of the current concept of depression, physicians have transitioned their definition of science to match new scientific practices over the last century.

To make the claim, as many do, that depression is a *real* disease—just like other diseases such as cancer or heart disease—is to make a historically contingent, political statement. Modern psychiatrists, anxious to distance themselves from a time when psychiatrists talked about penis envy and Oedipal conflicts, make special efforts to insist that mental diseases are brain diseases and are treated with real medical interventions (medicines).[13] The insistence on the real nature of depression has been a part of psychiatrists' professional redefinition in the second half of the twentieth century. A century ago, psychiatrists would not have needed to insist that insanity was a real disease—anyone who visited insane asylums could see that these individuals were really and truly ill. Now, when individuals' treatment for psychiatric illness is generally invisible, psychiatrists reassure themselves and their patients that depression counts as a serious illness, that patients deserve treatment—and that psychiatrists deserve respect for uncovering this important disease.

Psychiatrists and other activists for depression also emphasize the global prevalence of depression, stressing the worldwide burden of morbidity and mortality from this illness. Yet these claims about depression's ubiquity have emerged in the context of depression's incorporation into American—and increasingly global—mass culture. The language of depression as an explanation for Americans' failure to be happy brings with it not only an external solution—medication—but also a ready and growing market for the pharmaceutical industry. Depression's success as a disease concept—as measured by marketing figures in the pharmaceutical industry as well as research productivity within psychiatry—is a testament to how well the concept fit within mass culture in the second half of the twentieth century, particularly the increasing tendency to identify a problem with a consumer solution. And American assumptions about depression, especially its commercial significance, are being exported (along with other elements of American mass culture) to other countries.

Finally, researchers, physicians, and a significant population of patients and patient advocates emphasize depression as a major health problem that affects women. The claims about depression's greater prevalence in women have been entirely contingent on ongoing assumptions about gender and treatment of women patients—assumptions that helped to construct clinical trials and diagnostic criteria. But it is a major leap to move from decades of research in depression—research based on social and cultural assumptions about women—to the claim that depression must be linked to some unique feature of women's brains. Some have argued that psychiatry's propensity to see differences between men and women in psychiatric diagnoses indicates ongoing sexism.[14] Yet while many diseases diagnosed in the past in predominantly female patient populations were often the result of enforced patriarchal authority from physicians, the story of depression is more complicated than one of bias or simple sexist views of women. Instead, there has been something about the diagnosis of depression that has captured the energy and efforts of women researchers and women patients, advocates who strongly believe that increased diagnosis and treatment of depression in women helps women achieve more in their lives.[15]

This book explores the emergence of depression as a specific category of illness from early-twentieth-century views of nervousness and insanity to the introduction of SSRIs for *DSM*-defined depression in the late 1980s and early 1990s. For this analysis, I focus on two main areas in which the emergence of depression has been most critical: medical journals (especially the *American Journal of Psychiatry*) and popular magazines.[16] While other areas of both medical practice and popular culture could contribute perspective to this problem, a view from the professional and popular periodicals allows us to see major changes over the twentieth century, particularly in the role of depression and the shifting language of mental disease and its context.

I have also chosen to focus this analysis on the twentieth century and the emergence of a specific diagnostic category for depression because the disease has had such important social, professional, and economic implications over this time period. It is possible to uncover descriptions of depression and depressive symptoms over the whole course of human history. Indeed, surveys such as the encyclopedic one produced by Stanley Jackson illustrate the similarities and differences of expressions of depression across different times and cultures.[17] But what is important about our current diagnosis of depression is not what it has in common with ancient theories, but rather what is specific about the function of the diagnosis in the twentieth century. Modern depression has helped to shape psychiatry through major treatment upheavals, facilitated the merging of interests between pharmaceutical companies and professionals, justified the construction of research infrastructure, and helped to shape everyday experiences for a large number of American women. Depression as we know it now is important to American psychiatry and society, and this book explores this recent specific history.

In making the argument that depression (as we know it now) says more about our culture and our society than our mental states, I am not arguing that it does not exist. As a practicing psychiatrist, I frequently encounter seriously ill individuals who clearly suffer from depression and need treatment. But the modern label of depression does not just refer to those very sick people; it also refers to individuals who are not sure what they want in their lives, are not entirely happy, are in difficult home or work situations, or who would like to feel better than they do. Are the experiences of all these people the product of the same disease as the one afflicting people who have to be in the hospital because they cannot eat or sleep and constantly think about suicide?

This book traces the growth of depression as an object of medical study and as a consumer commodity over the twentieth century and illustrates how and why depression came to be such a huge medical, social, and cultural phenomenon. I do not make any attempt to determine who is sick and who is not, nor do I make suggestions about which individuals should get treatment. I do not advance a conspiracy theory about either professionals or industries. Instead, this is a story of well-meaning individuals and their desire to help others—but it is also a story of the contingencies in scientific and medical theory and practice.[18] A diagnosis can be a powerful tool to help others, but it can also obscure personal, social, cultural, and economic factors that are part of how people live their lives. Our modern diagnosis of depression may sound scientific and compelling, but that does not mean that it should be mindlessly applied or that it should go unquestioned. This book addresses the key questions of how the diagnosis of depression was developed, how it has been used, and how we should further question its application in American society.

Chapter 1

Prelude to Depression

Current researchers in the area of depression often emphasize the long history of the disease and cite representations from the past from figures such as Hippocrates, Richard Burton, and Shakespeare to illustrate that this has been an ancient and important problem for humankind.[1] Yet these past images of depression did not lead directly to our modern diagnosis of depression. If we look at early-twentieth-century psychiatry and neurology textbooks, for example, we find that depression (or melancholia) was not a major focus of professional attention. Indeed, these early texts do not include a disease category of depression at all. Further, Americans only a century ago would have assumed that depression was an economic problem, not a psychiatric illness. So how did we get our modern diagnosis of depression, and how did it develop its modern meaning in American culture?

The history of psychiatric illness—as with the history of any illness—is not just about symptoms or treatment, it is about the scientific and medical context in which practitioners viewed symptoms and outlined definitions of disease, as well as the social and cultural contexts in which physicians and patients interacted around diagnosis and treatment. Ancient traditions of melancholia did not directly evolve into our modern, criteria-based concept of depression. On the contrary, melancholia as originally described within the context of Hippocratic (humoral) theories of the body and disease had little relevance to American psychiatrists by the time the profession was organized in the mid-nineteenth century.[2]

American practitioners of mental medicine in the early twentieth century faced significant professional challenges with vague disease concepts, competition for patients, and an unclear path within medicine's move toward science in the first decades of the century. Readers of popular magazines increasingly encountered representations of nervousness, as well as insanity, that suggested that Americans were vulnerable to mental ailments. Although depression was not a specific concept within either medical or popular magazine literatures in the first half of the century, depression emerged in the second half of the twentieth century as a solution to the problems in the professions of mental medicine and took root within a growing American consumer culture.

Medical Context

In the first half of the twentieth century, two main groups of physicians engaged in the description, study, and treatment of diseases of the mind and brain.[3] Psychiatrists, whose specialty arose in the mid-nineteenth century around the care of individuals in institutions, focused much of their effort on the seriously ill (or insane, the accepted technical term of the time).[4] Neurologists, who began their specialty in sophisticated late-nineteenth-century medical markets in New York City and Philadelphia, described and promoted a variety of nervous diseases that could be cared for through office visit interventions.[5] The social settings in which psychiatrists and neurologists practiced shaped their assumptions about illness, their ideas about the role of symptoms, and their methods of treatment. And these social settings shaped how, when, and why practitioners addressed melancholic or depressive symptoms.

For example, in 1901 Binghamton State Hospital's Assistant Physician Cecil MacCoy published a case report of a twenty-eight-year-old man "of intemperate habits" who was admitted to the hospital after he attempted suicide. MacCoy described the patient's history as similar to other "alcoholic melancholics," and his first eight months of treatment were characterized by "ordinary" melancholic experiences including visual and auditory hallucinations, persecutory delusions, and poor appetite. The patient then progressed to a stuporous state and eventually had to be fed by a tube, while his muscles needed stimulation with electrical current. With the perseverance of the hospital staff, the patient was finally—close to four years from the onset of his symptoms—able to get out of bed and talk about his experiences. MacCoy's article was illustrated with two pictures: the first of an ill-appearing, bed-bound patient; the second an alert, well-dressed man in a gentlemanly posture, holding a book. MacCoy's case report indicated that the patient was soon to be discharged and that his prognosis was good.[6] MacCoy's lengthy contact with this melancholic patient was typical for the time period, not necessarily because of the patient's signs or symptoms but because of the setting in which he received his care.

But early-twentieth-century neurologists had significantly different experiences with patients. Although many neurologists saw individuals who presented with what we would today characterize as psychiatric complaints, neurologists treated them for a different set of symptoms and in different settings than their contemporary psychiatric colleagues. Early in his career, influential New York neurologist Smith Ely Jelliffe published several accounts of his first dispensary practice.[7] In 1903, Jelliffe reported that he saw 1,780 patients over the previous year, 30 of whom were suffering from melancholia. In addition to this small number of cases of melancholia, he saw some hysteria, convulsive disorders, and lots of neurasthenia—as he explained, "Neurasthenia is par excellence the disease of dispensary patients." Jelliffe's encounter with patients was at a much more rapid pace that MacCoy's—Jelliffe obviously saw a large number of patients over the year, and he did not provide information about specific stories or follow-up on cases. Jelliffe's patients walked in, received some sort of assistance, and walked out.[8]

The contrast between the experiences of these two young practitioners—MacCoy in the hospital and Jelliffe in the dispensary—was typical for the differences between psychiatrists and neurologists in the first decades of the twentieth century. In this time period, psychiatrists and neurologists practiced in fairly well defined spaces with poorly defined disease concepts. Psychiatrists saw seriously disordered persons with varying symptoms whose main problem was that they were unable to leave the structure of the hospital. Neurologists saw patients with troubling yet mysterious physical and emotional symptoms in outpatient settings and attempted to provide them relief by addressing those symptoms. Neither specialty defined itself in terms of specific disease categories or specific therapies.

American psychiatrists in the early part of the century framed their understanding of mental disease in the context of their hospital care. Although they borrowed conceptualizations first from Berlin professor Wilhelm Griesinger and later from German psychiatrist and nosologist Emil Kraepelin, American psychiatrists emphasized the importance of the local environment in describing forms of mental illness.[9] Thus, for example, while Hudson River State Hospital Superintendent Charles Pilgrim reported on the experiences of Griesinger and Kraepelin, he attributed differences in his patients' diagnoses to environmental effects rather than a failure of diagnosis.[10] Most American psychiatrists used Kraepelin's concept of the disease of manic-depressive insanity (or psychosis), a form characterized by both melancholia and mania.[11] Yet the significance of melancholia—as symptom, complaint, description—varied widely in psychia-trists' accounts of their patients.[12]

While American psychiatrists described the many presentations of insanity in hospitals—including melancholic manifestations—neurologists were more preoccupied with the best-known American nervous ailment: neurasthenia. Originally described in the 1870s by American neurologist George M. Beard, neurasthenia appeared to be the quintessential problem for a nation captured by its need to rush around with new technologies.[13] Though neurasthenia was beginning to wane in American medical literatures by the second and third decades of the twentieth century, it was a significant touchstone for practitioners in the field as an illness around which they could define their professional activities.[14] Melancholia sometimes appeared with neurasthenia, and occasionally neurologists named a condition they identified as "simple depression," though it was never well defined, nor was its relationship with neurasthenia clearly established.[15]

Since disease concepts were not well defined, most practitioners focused on the need to alleviate symptoms—among them, depression. But though both psychiatrists and neurologists emphasized the relief of symptoms, symptom relief meant different things in different treatment settings. In general, psychia-trists followed the tradition of allopathic treatment and treated symptoms of illness through inducing their opposite (for example, providing laxatives for patients complaining of constipation).[16] This approach toward mental illness led to a number of creative therapies (some of which could be dangerous) in the first half of the century, including gastric lavage for indigestion and constipation, as well as measures to activate lethargic patients or calm agitated patients.[17] The goal of treatment was to help patients leave the hospital.

Although psychiatrists focused on the hospital context, neurologists in the first part of the century treated depressive symptoms in the same way as other types of symptoms, particularly with an emphasis on rest and feeding.[18] Patients who consulted neurologists might have been offered reassurance or were encouraged to engage in moderate physical activity.[19] Maintenance of sleep was a priority for patients with mental disease, and physicians agreed that drugs for sleep could be quite helpful.[20] Neurologists also offered "psycho-logic treatment" or "psychotherapy," which involved anything from discussion of the patient's personal habits to the minutiae of his or her thoughts.[21] For the most part, neurologists focused on helping patients back on a road toward sufficient health, particularly to avoid having to be hospitalized.

One major difference between outpatient treatment of depressive symp-toms and hospital-based treatment was in the distinction between normal states and disease states requiring treatment. While psychiatrists in hospitals illustrated their patients' severe disturbances, neurologists' accounts of their patients' complaints were much closer to normal. As Meyer Solomon, a professor of neurology from the Chicago College of Medicine, pointed out in the *Chicago Medical Record* in 1915, everyone was susceptible to the blues, and the remedy was simple: "The lesson to be learned from this is as follows: Lead an active but varied life. Live a full life. Avoid narrow living, getting into ruts, monotony and rigid routine. Give all your better energies a satisfactory outlet. Unfold and give full rein to all those feelings and qualities which are worthy and demand exercise. Variety is indeed the spice of life."[22] Solomon's practice advice could have been taken as information to give patients—or possibly advice to the practitioners.

But though psychiatrists and neurologists focused on the treatment of symptoms (some that were more severe than others), leaders within the professions were concerned about the relationship between symptoms and disease definitions. While our early-twenty-first-century diagnoses are based on symptom criteria, that did not seem to be a valid possibility for early-twentieth-century psychiatrists or neurologists. Clarence Farrar, an influential psychiatrist at the Sheppard and Enoch Pratt Hospital and the Johns Hopkins University, argued in 1905 that classifying mental illness based on symptoms would be "equivalent to saying that a patient whose chief objective symptom may be labored breathing is suffering from dyspnoea, and letting the diagnosis rest there."[23] Symptoms, many insisted, were only the outward manifestations of bodily pathology. In line with medical knowledge of the time that disease followed discrete lesion or disturbance in physiology, psychiatrists argued that they needed to find true etiology for insanity before putting too much stock in classification.[24] As Johns Hopkins Hospital internist Lewellys Barker explained in 1914, psychiatrists needed a great deal more information about normal and abnormal states of mind in order to form more objective classification schemes.[25]

Indeed, mental medicine practitioners in the first half of the century seldom defined diseases more distinctly than with names, nor did the lack of specific disease definitions appear to be a major professional concern.[26] Instead, neurologists and psychiatrists in the early decades of the century became increasingly defensive about their specialties' use of science at a time in which the application of the laboratory to clinical medicine was bearing dividends.[27] In the first few decades of the century, psychiatrists responded to calls for science in medicine by beginning to articulate the importance of psychiatric intervention beyond the confines of the hospital.[28] Some psychiatrists and neurologists also worked on basic laboratory interventions, including pathological anatomy.[29] But while the disconnect between mental medicine and the rest of medical care was discussed in the early years of the century, the increasing calls for laboratory science and specific disease-based interventions significantly affected psychiatry and neurology by midcentury.

By the 1930s and 1940s, a number of shifts began to take place within the professions as both neurologists and psychiatrists attempted to make their specialties more scientific, though each interpreted science in medicine in a different way. Most neurologists, while still collaborating with psychiatrists in the 1934 formation of the American Board of Psychiatry and Neurology, became more interested in structural nerve problems and embraced the microscope and mechanical means to visualize the nervous system.[30] Psychiatrists began to question the traditional orientation of psychiatry, and suggested that the profession needed to shift in the direction of psychiatric research.[31] Three areas in particular appeared to be appropriate for new psychiatric efforts by this time: an increased focus on psychoanalytic theory, more emphasis on somatic therapies, and more tightly constructed disease nosologies. Depression as a concept had an increasingly prominent role within these areas.

Melancholia had a particular significance for those practitioners interested in psychoanalysis, especially those who followed Sigmund Freud's lead from his 1917 essay *Mourning and Melancholia*.[32] Within a psychoanalytic framework, symptoms represented access points to patients' unconscious conflicts. There was little consensus in the early part of the century on what might cause melancholic symptoms, although by the 1920s and 1930s psychoanalysts developed an elaborate set of theories around this based on the idea that depression represented introjected aggression toward a lost object.[33] For analysts, depression provided an opportunity to engage in rich interpretive possibilities around patients' drives and conflicts. Early enthusiasts emphasized, though, that psychoanalytic explanatory theories were more than just creative ways of reading patient conflicts—they were actually part of a scientific examination of the patient, analogous to a physical examination. In fact, the careful analysis of cases could help psychoanalysts determine the difference between a psychogenic depression and a depression that was part of a manic-depressive psychosis (their fixations would be different).[34]

At the same time that some psychiatrists (and a few neurologists) were working out psychoanalytic theories, others were increasingly focused on somatic treatments to treat mental illness (though sometimes with a psychoanalytic frame of reference).[35] By the 1930s, a number of psychiatrists began to apply remedies to patients' bodies that were specific to groups of psychiatric symptoms. In the course of exploring these treatments, psychiatrists focused on more specific diagnostic entities, particularly manic-depressive psychosis and schizophrenia. During this time period, there were few proposed medications for depressive illness.[36] By far the most dramatic and widespread somatic (applied to the body) therapies between the 1930s and the 1950s were shock therapies and lobotomy. Shock therapies, which included insulin shock, metrazol, and electric shock, were used to treat agitation, improve patients' thought processes, and help patients engage in more productive psycho-therapy.[37] Metrazol and electric shock in particular appeared specifically to benefit patients with depressive symptoms, while lobotomy was used for patients with behavior problems and prolonged hospitalizations.[38] Through the enthusiastic embrace of both psychoanalysis and somatic therapies by the 1940s, American psychiatrists were in a position to put more energy into the symptom of depression.

But depression was still not a diagnosis, though psychiatrists (and some neurologists) by the 1930s began to participate in the broader movement within the American professions toward a more systematic accounting of their disease classifications.[39] Physicians' increasing interest in classification provided the opportunity to adopt another tool of modern science: statistics.[40] In 1928, the New York Academy of Medicine convened a conference with a number of medical organizations to discuss the need for more organized classification of medical illnesses and improved statistical tabulation of morbidity and mortality data. The National Conference on Nomenclature of Disease, led by public health reformer Haven Emerson, was founded as a result of this meeting, and participants in the conference engaged in a three-year project (funded by the Commonwealth Fund and several insurance companies) to develop a standardized nomenclature, which was finally published in 1933.[41] Both the American Psychiatric Association and the American Neurological Association were represented within this new nomenclature.

Though the authors of the 1933 classification system worked hard to include all possible categories of disease, the use of these categories in prac-tice was less clear, particularly with regard to mental disease. For example, Baltimore psychiatrist Leslie Hohman pointed out in 1937 that the diagnosis of manic-depressive psychosis did not fit well with how psychiatrists diagnosed and treated patients: "Either we have followed slavishly the manic-depressive doctrine and forcibly distorted cases to fit the mold; or, we have rejected the manic-depressive concept and have been tempted to throw overboard all the of the virtue of the idea of symptomatology, course and outcome. With the rejection we have reached for (a) *complete* psychogenesis or (b) brain disease explanation."[42] Psychiatrists studied different populations, found different symptoms, drew different diagnostic conclusions, and made different suppositions about the nature of psychiatric nosology during this time period, despite the availability of lists of possible diseases. Neurologists were even less invested in their own nosological systems and did not generally engage in major debate about the details.

Although psychiatrists invested time and energy on psychoanalytic concepts, somatic therapies, and disease nosologies, they remained vulnerable to ongoing criticism that their specialty was less than scientific. Some commented that psychoanalytic ideas, while broad in their possibilities, were perhaps too fuzzy to provide the scientific backbone for the specialty. Further, the somatic therapies, as useful as they were for some patients, were still linked primarily to the hospital setting—a setting that was increasingly problematic with the midcentury exposés of institutional treatment. Finally, the disease classification approach left open the question of how to define patients. The psychiatrists interested in a psychoanalytic approach toward patients argued that it was impossible to learn more about mental disease by grouping people into categories, while those who were interested in disease concepts argued that research into disease course and prognosis was critical to understand mental illness.

These issues all remained in the second half of the century, but the introduction of psychiatric medications organized psychiatric research and efforts toward a focus on specific diseases, particularly depression. Anxiety also led toward specific therapies and diagnoses in the second half of the century, but its connection to the psychoanalytic community through the terminology of neuroses may have limited its appeal to opponents of psychoanalysis in the 1960s and 1970s.[43] The concept of depression clearly relied on the influence of psychoanalytic theory, yet it was also an indication for somatic therapy. Further, as research into depression treatments continued in the 1960s and 1970s, depression provided a new model for constructing disease categories. Depression did not come out of nowhere, but rather represented a way for psychiatrists to solve professional problems—as well as problems for their patients—in the second half of the century.

Popular Accounts

Depression's success in the second half of the twentieth century relied both on its usefulness within physician writings as well as its resonance within American popular culture. Over the century there have been significant connections between medical understandings of mental disturbances and popular expressions of them—if nothing else, physicians have been contributors to both types of literature. But the flow of information has not been in just one direction. Instead, the discourse of mental illness in popular magazines reflected both cultural and medical elements, while cultural assumptions in turn became incorporated into medical literature.[44] Writers for popular magazines made suggestions to physicians as well as to potential or actual patients. And physicians observed popular enthusiasm for specific concepts in their own literatures.[45] While psychiatrists, like other physicians, usually scorned publicity for their treatment efforts, they were certainly not adverse to trying to intervene in popular media in order to try to influence public opinion.[46]

Depression as an illness became meaningful to the American public because of the ways in which it addressed preexisting conflicts and issues within American culture, issues that can be traced in changes in popular magazine coverage in the first half of the twentieth century. During this time period, magazines circulated in greater and greater numbers, connecting communities of increasingly literate customers and instructing them with stories, advice, and advertisements.[47] In the general audience periodicals, Americans encountered discussions of both insanity (which afflicted only those in asylums) and nervousness (which could affect anyone). But after the first few decades of the century, popular descriptions of both nervousness and insanity gradually merged concerns about the two and promoted the idea that anyone could be afflicted with a mental illness. American readers who accepted responsibility for maintaining their emotional health were introduced to the idea that mental health needed to be pursued in a specific way. Mental hygiene was the first major consumer product in popular literature and prepared the way for increasingly consumerized approaches toward mental health and illness in the second half of the century.[48] Finally, readers increasingly encountered the idea that Americans were both prone to illness and likely to pioneer in treatments.

Readers of popular magazines in the early twentieth century could not have turned many pages before encountering some kind of description of nervousness or neurasthenia. Physicians sometimes wrote these accounts, but also interested laypersons and journalists sounded the alarm about the perceived extent of nervous illness in the United States.[49] Nervous illness appeared so prevalent in the first half of the twentieth century that writers sometimes complained that people were too quick to attribute all their problems to their nerves.[50] Popular magazine accounts both described nervousness in others and suggested nervousness in readers by addressing them directly in the second person.[51] As Dr. Henry Smith Williams wrote in *Good Housekeeping* in 1914, "But now, at last, too greatly imposed on, the ganglia of the sympathetic system make a protest that is heard at the headquarters in the brain. Hence your head-aches, your indigestion, your feeling of apprehension and depression, your wakefulness at night and lassitude by day, your irritability and 'nervousness' in general."[52] Popular enthusiasm for discussions of nervousness expanded well beyond magazines, and physician advice books appeared on the market to help nervous sufferers through their difficult times.[53]

Readers of popular magazines were encouraged to see themselves (or their loved ones) as possible sufferers of nervousness in general or neurasthenia in particular. But insanity, which was also a frequent topic in popular literature in the early twentieth century, was a much more foreign and distant concept. Instead of presentations on insanity from the sufferer's point of view, most focused on the doctor's perspective.[54] Indeed, as a physician explained in 1900, one problem was that "writers still treat insanity as an entity apart from its bearings on the average mind and its evolutionary history. The word 'insanity,' or 'lunatic,' is no doubt largely responsible for this, suggesting popularly, as it does, a distinct class of persons—a type of being as unlike ourselves as a Martian might be fancied to be."[55] While accounts of insanity shifted consider-ably over the decades, the concept of insanity as something completely different and separate from normal experience lingered. As another physician pointed out in 1936, "Insanity is a horrible word. Most of us think of it as something loathsome and mysterious; a taint in the blood; hopeless; incurable."[56] Insanity continued to appear profoundly different from the experiences of most people, and physicians, as well as laypersons, helped to continue that separation.

Yet there were possible connections between the two, as some (especially psychiatrists) suggested that unchecked neurosis might lead to insanity. Thus everyday neurotic symptoms became dangerous warning signs that should not be ignored. One physician argued that too many people were striving for a higher status career than their abilities warranted, and were becoming too nervous through their education.[57] The results were not just decreased work productivity but also the substantial risk for insanity. Lay writers also echoed physician warnings about the need to avoid overwork or excessive emotional displays, as well as the need to engage in good digestive habits, since uncontrolled neurasthenia could lead to insanity.[58] In these accounts, insanity represented a frightening and unknown worst possible consequence. Writers did not illustrate cases of people who were first nervous and then became insane, but the threat was there that nervous sufferers might become insane if they did not control their nervousness. Further, this ongoing risk suggested that readers might need a physician's advice—sooner if not later.

The boundaries between nervousness and insanity began to blur as psychiatrists became authorities for larger and larger segments of the population in the 1930s and 1940s. By this time, psychiatrists were not only the heads of mental institutions, they were also the arbiters of selective service screening, cultural authorities regarding human nature, and the purveyors of new therapies. While the psychiatric hospital remained a foreign and frightening place, representations of mental illness by the middle of the century appeared less tied to institutions. Psychiatrists recognized that they needed to distance themselves from their older reputation as custodians of insane asylums and began to discourage the use of the term "insane."[59] Psychiatrists probably did not actively plot to get themselves more publicity in popular magazines, but as a profession they actively touted their expertise in ever-expanding areas.

Psychiatric successes during World War II helped to convince the public that psychiatry had something to offer to regular citizens.[60] Popular magazine authors at the beginning of the war emphasized the extent to which psychiatrists were involved in screening applicants for the war.[61] During the war, popular commentators extolled the efforts of psychiatrists to quickly return soldiers with war neuroses to the front.[62] Further, authors emphasized that psychiatric casualties of war were just as real and significant as physical casualties and did not reflect on soldiers' general sanity.[63] As one doctor was quoted in an article in *Recreation*, "Soldiers suffering from combat fatigue are just nervously sick, not diseased, and therefore no stigma of mental illness can be attached to their condition."[64] Psychiatrists also weighed in on the deleterious effects of war on the civilian population's mental health.[65] Thus through their experiences with the war, psychiatrists became seen more as medical doctors treating war-related injuries than just authorities over an insane population in a hospital.

Not only did psychiatrists appear more like general doctors, but also their treatments—especially new interventions such as narcosynthesis—appeared to be more like those of other physicians. Psychiatrists during World War II argued that men who returned from combat unable to speak or to explain their terror would rapidly improve if they could talk about their experiences. This belief in the power of a talking cure was clearly driven by psychoanalytic belief in working through conflicts. But though World War II psychiatrists wanted patients to talk things through, they did not have the years of contact with patients to get to the combat issues. Instead, American psychiatrists gave Sodium Pentothal to soldiers who came to them with symptoms of "war neurosis" or "exhaustion." Under the influence of Sodium Pentothal, the soldiers were able to talk about their experiences, do some quick work on resolving their conflicts, and then return to the front.[66]

American experiences during World War II helped to increase familiarity with psychiatrists even for those who had never gone to see a mental health professional.[67] As a popular commentator pointed out in a 1944 *Collier's* article, more people than ever before had become aware of psychiatric work both through popular media coverage of war neuroses and through personal contact with the selective service screening. In this context, Americans were confronted with the possibility that anyone could be diagnosed with a psychiatric ailment or even rejected for war service for this reason. As the author in *Collier's* pointed out, however, psychiatric ailments no longer had overtones of madness: "To be diagnosed as a psychoneurotic does not mean a person is crazy or insane. The neurotic is generally a maladjusted and oversensitive individual."[68] Popular magazine authors emphasized that psychiatric symptoms were possible in everyday life, not a necessary indicator of the need to be locked away in an asylum.

As early-twentieth-century readers encountered mental disease in the pages of their favorite magazines, they also encountered advice about how to proceed if they (or someone they knew) suffered from such an illness. This advice sometimes consisted of instruction to seek out a medical professional for treatment. But often writers in popular magazines urged readers to take matters into their own hands and correct their problems rather than rely on experts. By the 1930s, American readers were increasingly presented with a specific vision of how to achieve mental health, the vision actively promoted by the mental hygiene movement. As activists within the movement self-consciously attempted to sell their vision to the American public, the language of mental health and illness became imbued with the language of consumerism. Initially, the opportunities for consumption appeared around issues of nervousness. By the middle of the century, though, the concepts broadened to include all mental health.

Most descriptions of treatment for nervousness during this time period included commonsense interventions such as appropriate balance between work and rest, attention to activities outside oneself, and adequate nutrition.[69] Although physicians provided information on nervousness, they did not necessarily tout the importance of physician interventions. In fact, they occasionally warned readers against going to the doctor for a quick fix: "Patients are unwilling to follow a definite, reasonable, carefully thought-out plan of life, and beg for a specific, for some drug that can be taken in teaspoonful doses three times a day, to serve instead of temperance, soberness, and chastity."[70] Popular writers (including physician contributors) often argued that individuals should help themselves instead of only depending on physicians.[71]

But self-help did not necessarily mean that individuals were on their own. In the first decades of the century, the Emmanuel Movement in Boston, a group of religious and psychiatric experts who announced that they would help individuals help themselves, received a great deal of popular attention. The Emmanuel Movement was directed by the Reverend Samuel McComb, who argued that "suggestion"—a pattern of repeating self-affirming statements while in a relaxed state—could reduce nervousness, particularly in American women.[72] The Emmanuel Movement's emphasis on suggestion was part of a larger cultural discussion about the connection between nervousness and a lack of self-control. Some emphasized the need for self-control to overcome emotional overindulgence and nervous physical habits such as twitches, while others stressed the importance of achieving control over the environment.[73] At the same time that nervous sufferers needed to take control of themselves, they also needed to avoid being selfish and self-absorbed.[74] With self-control, as the Reverend McComb and others argued, nervous sufferers would have no need for physician interventions.[75]

But for readers in the first half of the century, it was not enough merely to avoid nervousness or other forms of mental illness; instead, they needed to actively pursue mental health. The most organized system of mental health education and prevention in the United States was the mental hygiene movement, based initially on the experiences of Clifford Beers, whose 1908 book, *A Mind That Found Itself*, helped to spur interest in mental health.[76] Advocates inside and outside the movement engaged in the vital effort to spread the word about mental health based on the idea that effective education could actually prevent insanity. These educational efforts took place in schools, in workplaces, and through the pages of popular magazines. For example, well-known psychiatrist Karl Menninger wrote a series in *Ladies' Home Journal* for more than a year about the importance of health at home and proper family relationships.[77] Mental health advocates focused attention on mental disease prevention through the promotion of good health habits and the avoidance of bad ones.[78]

While mental hygiene activists promoted what appeared to be fairly commonsense ideas about health, they were aware that not everyone would necessarily accept their advice. George Pratt, the medical director for the Massachusetts Society for Mental Hygiene, argued in 1924 that psychiatrists needed to "sell" the idea of mental hygiene to the public with the analogy of selling merchandise. He explained that the public needed to know that they needed mental hygiene; in other words, the demand had to be created in order to appropriately sell the product. Pratt pointed out that most of the public could not comprehend the jargon about mental illness that was generally used by physicians, and he advocated using simplified language to sell ideas.[79]

At the same time that physician writers and mental health advocates educated the public about the concepts of mental health and illness, they also provided a vocabulary with which commentators could frame their concerns. Americans were increasingly aware of and used psychological language in the years after World War II.[80] By the 1950s, many Americans had access to the language of mental symptoms, from the popular versions of Freudian concepts to the language surrounding the increasing use of treatments such as shock therapy. This education not only gave consumers of popular media the language to describe mental symptoms, it also allowed them access to a broad vocabulary to describe other kinds of problems. In addition, the language of mental disorders significantly helped psychiatrists as they continued to expand their presence in the public arena. The sense of urgency with which popular magazine commentators worked to sell the idea of mental hygiene was transferred in the second half of the century to another great threat to American health: depression.

In the first decades of the twentieth century, America appeared to be in danger from a multitude of external and internal ailments. Public health officials worried about immigrants bringing in infectious diseases.[81] Eugenics enthusiasts deplored the lamentable state of the nation's intelligence and warned of the dire consequences of the reproduction of inferior stock.[82] Many worried about how the United States would fare in competition or relationship with other countries. And all expressed both enthusiasm and doubt about the rollicking speed with which Americans were encountering the new trappings of modern civilization.[83] Both nervous disease and insanity were evidence of America's precarious position, and the ways in which the country dealt with these issues appeared to be a barometer of American progress.

Physicians and lay writers in the popular literature in the first half of the twentieth century agreed that nervousness was a particular problem for Americans. As one physician observed in 1910, "Americanitis, nervous prostration, neurasthenia, whatever name one may prefer to use, is a condition produced by the failure of the nervous system to generate or impart its accustomed vigor to the organs, tissues, muscles, etc., depending on it for proper function."[84] Most assumed that the modern rush of civilization was increasing Americans' tendency to become nervous.[85] But while some commentators were concerned about American nervousness, others suggested that it was actually a by-product of American ingenuity, inventiveness, and boundless energy.[86] Physician William Sadler characterized the United States in 1925 in terms of a national desire to succeed: "As a nation, we drive ahead, trying to lead the world, to outrival everybody else. We have a mania for speed, thrills, excitement. We are victims of Americanitis."[87] Americanitis was thus both a precipitant of illness and a description of a particular intensity and desire to achieve. While some writers were more negative than others about the implications of Americanitis for the future of the nation, there was a definite overtone of American superiority in this condition.[88]

American propensity to nervousness might signal superior abilities, but American tendencies toward insanity could be a national threat. On the one hand, Americans reassured themselves that their national leaders did not tend toward insanity and compared them favorably to Europe's many past and present degenerate and insane rulers.[89] But while American conditions might be less dangerous than those in Europe, America was not immune to problems with insanity. Indeed, writers for popular magazines warned that the nation could be evaluated based on the state of its insane population, both in terms of their numbers and in terms of their humane treatment. As one writer explained, "Insanity is a delicate index of national ill-health."[90] Popular writers regularly reported that modern conditions—particularly war, immigration, the shift of the population to cities, and increasing racial mixes within the cities—were causing the rates of insanity to increase.[91]

Early in the century, many popular writers advocated eugenics methods to deal with the problem of insanity.[92] By the 1930s and 1940s, however, writers were significantly less likely to blame heredity and instead focused on the plight of the insane in mental hospitals.[93] Hospitals represented the locus for the most seriously mentally ill, a locus that was both horrifying in its condition and hopeful in the possibilities for scientific advancement. Scientist and popular writer Paul de Kruif profiled a number of "Men Fixing Life" in a *Ladies' Home Journal* article in 1932 in which he lauded the efforts of psychiatrists who were trying out specific somatic treatments for the insane, such as carbon dioxide and sodium amytal: "So after centuries of mere mysticism, of psychologizing, men are fixing at sick-brained people. Some day they'll empty asylums."[94] In the subsequent decade, popular writers enthusiastically described a variety of somatic interventions for insanity and proclaimed that psychiatrists had finally joined the remainder of the medical profession in terms of their abilities to help people.[95]

These treatments for insanity had a significant effect on the portrayals of mental illness in popular magazines. Instead of just describing insanity, a general concept that often implied bizarre and frightening behaviors, popular commentators began to discuss specific mental illnesses with an emphasis on their treatments.[96] With the introduction of insulin coma therapy, metrazol, and electric shock therapies in the late 1930s and early 1940s, popular press coverage of insanity began to mention the diagnosis of dementia praecox, or schizophrenia. Popular writers focused on the devastations of schizophrenia and the difficulties in treating that illness, rather than just the general problem of insanity.[97] Most commentators explained that schizophrenia was not the only type of illness that afflicted patients in mental hospitals, but they did emphasize how difficult it had been to treat prior to the introduction of new, promising somatic treatments. While some cautioned that the new treatments for schizophrenia might not turn out to be as effective as they originally appeared, authors were still enthusiastic about insulin shock and metrazol because psychiatry finally had new tools with which to battle mental ailments.[98] Further, the new somatic therapies had implications for what some believed to be a weakness in the profession. As one writer reported in *Forum* in 1939, the "grip of psychoanalysis on popular imagination has been a chronic source of irritation to the clinical psychiatrists, the men who, unlike the disciples of Freud, work day in and out with [people with schizophrenia and manic depression]. They feel that Freud, a neurologist, has played leapfrog with scientific method in jumping from neurosis to psychosis." Thus the successes of insulin and metrazol shock would allow psychiatrists to throw out Freud's ideas.[99]

While the presence of nervousness might signal American superiority, American psychiatrists' triumph over major mental illness was another way to celebrate the national character. The popular magazine coverage of new treatments for insanity emphasized the exciting scientific work being applied to these severe illnesses. Although writers commented that schizophrenia was a serious illness that often resulted in institutionalization, popular writers in the 1930s and 1940s stressed the miracles of science in helping to treat individuals with schizophrenia. By midcentury, mental illness was not only a problem, it was also an opportunity for American professionals to demonstrate their ability to solve major problems. At the time that medications were introduced in the 1950s, Americans were poised to accept not only the treatment but also the diagnosis of psychiatry's latest challenge, depression.

By midcentury, American psychiatrists had a broad but awkward set of problems for which they had claimed responsibility. Social psychiatrists, including psychoanalytically inspired leaders of the field, emphasized that it was psychiatry's mission to bring improved mental health to the world. Psychiatrists increasingly occupied outpatient practices, taking care of neurotic

patients as neurologists gradually abandoned diseases for which there was
no visible pathology in favor of the care of patients with structural lesions
of the nervous system. Yet psychiatrists also continued to be in charge of the
large mental hospitals that garnered increasingly bad press in the 1950s.[100]
Midcentury psychiatrists made grand claims about their ability to improve
society, yet a significant gap appeared between their promises and the sickest
of their patients inside psychiatric institutions.[101] When medications appeared
on the scene in the 1950s and 1960s, many in the field grasped them as new
possibilities to help psychiatry become like other medical specialties with
medication treatments.

By the end of World War II, a substantial portion of the American public
had been exposed to ideas about mental illness and its treatment, as well
as major psychological terminology relating to the increasing circulation of
Freudian concepts. Psychiatrists had more or less established themselves
as authorities over mental problems, which included older concepts of
nervousness and insanity and the newer midcentury ideas of anxiety and
schizophrenia. Most Americans appeared to accept—based on the assumptions
by popular magazine writers—that mental phenomena were important to track
for individual and national health.

Yet at midcentury there was not yet a clearly defined need for specific
psychiatric intervention for depression, though there was professional and
popular discussion about national and individual anxiety.[102] Though Americans were anxious, they were not necessarily unhappy, especially during
the post–World War II boom years. By the late 1970s, though, unhappiness
appeared to be a major national problem, and its solution was presented as
increasing diagnosis and treatment of depression. The market for individual
mental health that emerged in the first half of the century expanded enormously
in the second half of the century—depression became both a commodity to
invest in (prevention and treatment in the name of national health) and a
problem in urgent need of a market solution (medications, therapy, marketed
self-help techniques). Depression did not emerge in the second half of the
century as a full-blown market phenomenon—it emerged in the context of
existing markets for personal and national mental health that had evolved in
the first half of the century. And depression as a disease to treat, define, and
research helped American psychiatrists as they struggled to redefine their
specialty in the second half of the twentieth century.

Chapter 2

The Expanding Diagnosis of Depression

In 1974, Jonathan Cole, chair of Temple University's Department of Psychiatry, reflected on recent treatment breakthroughs and research in depression in a special issue in the *American Journal of Psychiatry*. Cole explained that "from the psychiatrist's viewpoint only, depression is an exceedingly satisfactory disease. It is comforting, in this day of existential doubt and psychosocial malaise, to have an illness that is quite treatable and that is recognized by almost everyone as a real illness demanding real treatment."[1] Cole was enthusiastic that psychiatry finally had a "real illness" and a successful treatment for it, particularly because the "psychosocial malaise" of the time had been affecting the profession, too. Although depression was by no means the most severe illness psychiatrists were grappling with at the time, it assumed a larger and larger role in the medical literature through the 1970s. In the 1980s, depression was frequently described as the "common cold" of mental illness, and psychiatrists encouraged family practitioners to diagnose and treat it in their patients. By the 1990s, depression was one of the most common research topics in the psychiatric literature.

As historian and psychopharmacologist David Healy has persuasively argued, the idea of depression as a specific disease emerged with the introduction of medications for psychiatric problems in hospitals in the 1950s and beyond.[2] But medications did not just shape practice through selection and treatment of depressive symptoms. In addition, the increasing focus on depressive symptoms in the second half of the century helped to catalyze a major shift in psychiatric self-definition. This process was not inevitable. When the first psychiatric medications were introduced in the 1950s, they were primarily used to help calm agitation. Medications could have continued in that role, the way that other somatic interventions had been used earlier in the century—without organization of the field around the treatments. But medications appeared on the psychiatric scene at a critical moment in the profession's history, a time when a small but growing number of psychiatric researchers were increasingly dissatisfied with the social focus and grand claims of psychoanalytic leaders. These researchers seized upon the idea of treating mental illness with medications and used it to launch new ways of defining treatments, conceptualizing patients, and organizing disease classifications. Depression became a phenomenon around which professionals in the latter part of the twentieth century made claims about psychiatry's status as a scientific specialty.

Though psychiatrists stressed that depression was an example of a scientifically diagnosed and treated illness, they actively defined and redefined what counted as science. Between the 1950s and the 1980s, medication trials increasingly privileged academic researchers in larger groups working toward consensus over individual clinicians who claimed clinical experience. Academic researchers in turn looked to statistical manipulation of symptom frequency instead of narratives of illness. As symptoms became divorced from patient stories, psychiatrists and epidemiologists by the 1980s investigated general populations to uncover undiagnosed depression. For American psychiatry by the 1990s, depression was a glorious success as an illness: it was defined with specific criteria, had specific treatments (mostly medications), and appeared to affect large portions of the population. But depression's success came about not just with the use of scientific tools but also through the extent to which psychiatrists' definitions created the problem they credited themselves with being able to solve.

Defining Treatment

In the years after World War II, pharmaceutical companies grew rapidly in both scope and their relationships with physicians. New technologies of mass production had made broad-scale drug development, testing, and distribution possible for the first time. In the wake of American enthusiasm for penicillin and other remedies in the war years, pharmaceutical companies began to develop other compounds to test in a variety of settings.[3] Those clinical testing ventures led to frequent collaboration with physicians, including psychiatrists in charge of mental hospital patients. Psychiatric hospitals were logical places in which to test and track new medications, since the populations were large, there were few barriers to trying new treatments, and psychiatrists were eager to try to overcome public disfavor around conditions for the mentally ill inside hospitals.[4]

At midcentury, the psychiatric hospital environment could be chaotic, with behaviorally disturbed patients and overcrowded conditions.[5] In this setting, psychiatrists who used new medications began to measure success by whether patients appeared to improve, particularly in the lessened need for electroconvulsive therapy (ECT), or whether they could be advanced toward discharge.[6] Researchers, who ranged from individual clinicians trying out treatments to university-based investigators, increasingly commented on the effects of medication on patients who appeared depressed. Although a specific disease category of depression did not emerge until the 1970s, depressive symptoms gained increasing prominence with the expanding use of medications in psychiatric illness, and medication effects shaped how psychiatrists began to view patients.

Researchers who performed the initial clinical trials of psychiatric medication generally simply administered medications to a wide population of hospitalized patients and observed the results. In the 1950s, medications were not specifically designated for patients with particular diagnoses, and practitioners typically conceptualized most patients into one of two major categories: schizophrenia or manic-depressive psychosis. Chlorpromazine (Thorazine), which later become widely known as a medication for schizophrenia, was tested with good effect on patients with depressive symptoms.[7] Psychiatrists attempted to give medications to treat symptoms (not diagnoses) by opposites: some medications were used to calm agitation, while others appeared to give energy and motivation to those who looked depressed or slowed. For example, orphenadrine, a drug originally tested in parkinsonism, was found to have euphoric effects, and psychiatrists tried it out on patients with depressive symptoms.[8] Other investigators tested stimulants with the idea that depressed patients needed to be chemically roused out of their low state.[9] One of the first psychiatric medications used, iproniazid, was an antituberculosis medication that was noted to cause euphoria in patients with tuberculosis.[10]

Psychiatric investigators' reports of patient responses to medication in the 1950s were more descriptive than analytical.[11] Researchers used only percentages of patients within major categories of improved, partly improved, or not improved. Reports in the medical literature about medication effects tended to include case reports to best illustrate the dramatic improvement in the lives of the patients who received medications.[12] One of the first papers on the new antidepressant imipramine, which became the most widely known medication for depression over the subsequent two decades, measured outcome by looking at changes in four areas: subjective comfort, ward management, ability to go home, and social effectiveness. Improvement within each area was left to the researcher to define.[13]

During the 1950s, there were not major differences between the research methods of private practitioners and academic faculty, nor was research perceived to be better than clinical experience in demonstrating treatment efficacy. Indeed, Theodore Robie, a private practitioner in New Jersey who administered iproniazid (Marsalid) to large numbers of his patients, commented on the power of clinical experience compared to research investigation:

> During the 19 years that I have been giving ECT for melancholia, there have been many occasions when I have seen what appeared like a miracle as a severely depressed person emerged from despondency after a few treatments. But in the 33 years I have been practicing there has been no experience as satisfying as observing the occasional depressive who emerges from his despondency after a few days on Marsilid. To be sure there are very few that respond so quickly, but it is astounding to see when it does occur! It demonstrates *more convincingly than any statement any researcher can make*, what a remarkable chemical this is and how widespread will be its field of usefulness, once we have acquired the accurate methods of prescribing that are necessary to assure its safe application in each case.[14]

Academic researchers provided interesting and important information for practitioners, but authors in the professional literature often emphasized clinical experience rather than the evidence from research trials during this time period.

Both individual clinicians and investigative teams found medications helpful, but they defined medication efficacy in broad terms. What researchers did articulate clearly, however, was that medications such as imipramine helped patients who appeared depressed. As New York practitioner Benjamin Pollack explained about imipramine in 1959, "All research workers who used this drug initially were unanimous in the conclusion that, unlike many other psychopharmacological agents, it specifically affects depressive conditions and has very little effect on paranoid states or disturbed behavior, particularly in schizophrenics."[15] In later decades, researchers would begin to define patient diagnoses around their responses to medications.

While 1950s psychiatric researchers frequently enthused about the possibilities of medication, they seldom offered extensive descriptions of their research methodology or its potential limitations. Without much comment, psychiatrists in private practice and in hospitals provided the number of patients included in the study and usually mentioned the source of the patients (for example, hospital or outpatient clinics). Although researchers during the 1950s sometimes mentioned the general diagnosis of patients and how they came to be included in the trial (for example, consecutive admissions to the hospital), they never mentioned how much the patients knew about the trial or whether they had given consent to be included.[16]

By the 1960s, though, psychiatric researchers explicitly invoked the language of science to argue for better trials of medication and for improvement in the specialty's professional standing. But what it meant to make trials more scientific was open to some debate. Some researchers in academic centers began to form large collaborative research projects and to develop new assessment tools to use in research. But the move toward a basic science model of clinical research—with specific hypotheses, manipulation of variables, and attempts to remove human bias (in both researcher and subject)—was by no means immediately or widely accepted.[17] At the same time that some researchers were calling for better control of experiments to prove medical effectiveness of interventions, others insisted that clinical experience and case reports best represented science in psychiatry. When psychiatrists invoked "science," they did so within their own assumptions and expectations about what that meant.

Some investigators fairly early had begun to speculate about whether their methods of giving patients medications and noting improvement were objective enough to attribute all positive effects to medication alone. Robert Schopbach, a clinician at Henry Ford Hospital in Detroit, pointed out in 1958 the possibility of investigator bias in research, and emphasized that his trial of iproniazid was scientifically superior because he did not allow the use of "sales talk" prior to giving medication to his clinical subjects.[18] In 1959, Erwin Linn, from the Laboratory of Socio-Environmental Studies at the National Institute of Mental Health (NIMH), argued that it was difficult to sort out the differences between primary and side effects and to interpret patients' reports of improvement.[19] In response to these kinds of observations, some psychiatric researchers began to adopt the standard of the double-blind, placebo-controlled trial for study of medications. In this kind of trial, patients would be divided into different groups and given either a placebo (inactive agent) or an active drug; both the patients and the researchers were blind to which they were getting. Many researchers believed that this form of administering medication was more scientific since it allowed researchers to factor out the nonspecific effects of patients' high expectations inherent in research and treatment settings.[20]

Increasing numbers of potential medications became available in the 1960s, from imipramine to new monoamine oxidase inhibitors (MAOIs). Not only were medication studies more likely to include multiple drugs, but also researchers were more likely to use multiple sites for their studies and to select patients who might be responsive to the treatments. For example, the Massachusetts Mental Health Center collaborative project that was conducted in this time period employed a number of researchers from academic centers on the East Coast. In these large studies, researchers did not give medications to all patients, but rather specifically screened patients for depressive symptoms.[21]

Not all investigators agreed on the characteristics of the scientific method, though. Although some groups collaborated in large-scale, placebo-controlled trials, other researchers used case reports and psychoanalytic interpretations of small numbers of patients in order to employ some aspects of research methodology while preserving the authority of clinical experience.[22] One typical example of the flexible adaptation of research methodology in the 1960s was a study of 100 patients hospitalized in a state facility in Pennsylvania. The authors of the study randomized these patients into groups to compare response in symptoms to isocarboazid, nialamide, phenelzine, pheniprazine, and imipramine. The treating teams conducted symptom assessments before and after treatment and classified the patients into groups based on how many of the symptoms improved. Although these researchers clearly worked to try to address potential issues in their research methods, they invoked their "collaborative clinical experience" as the authority for the research.[23] For many researchers at the time, science could mean basic science (laboratory methods), clinical experience, psychoanalytic interpretation, or some combination of all of these.

Throughout these studies researchers made explicit assumptions that better research methods would yield better information about medication efficacy. But in the process, investigators changed the focus of the research from patients to medications. Instead of designing interventions around their patient populations, researchers selected patients in a way most likely to demonstrate medication effects. If patients did not respond the way they were expected to, maybe the patient selection—rather than the intervention—was wrong. For one researcher, the fact that his sample of depressed patients responded better to a medication that usually helped people with schizophrenia meant that his sample had been misdiagnosed.[24] Medications dictated diagnosis and patient selection, indeed to the point that medications began to shape how psychiatrists described their patients.

Defining Patients

Psychiatrists in the mid-twentieth century engaged in treatment of the seriously mentally ill in hospitals as well as increasing outpatient care of neuroses. But as psychiatry broadened its borders to include a wide range of mental illnesses, psychiatrists were not in full agreement about how to approach their patients. Although the distinction can become easily overblown, there was at least a rhetorical divide beginning in the early 1950s between psychiatrists with a more psychoanalytic and socially active focus and those with more of a research and biological focus.[25] In practice, psychiatrists could easily incorporate both psychoanalytic and biological approaches into the treatment of individual patients.[26] Yet the language of the psychoanalytic- and research-oriented psychiatrists differed in significant ways by the 1960s, particularly around their view of the doctor-patient relationship. In the light of psychiatric medication effects, some research psychiatrists began to actively reconsider how to understand, interact with, and define their patients—a process that led to increasing conflicts with their psychoanalytically oriented colleagues.

Psychiatric leaders who were heavily influenced by a psychoanalytic view of the world had long emphasized psychiatrists' roles as guardians of humanity with regard to the doctor-patient relationship and society as a whole.[27] But by the 1960s, a small but influential group of psychiatrists began to argue that psychiatrists needed to be less unique and more like other physicians. American Psychiatric Association (APA) medical director Walter Barton complained in 1962 that many psychiatrists did not behave like physicians—they did not interact with other physicians and did not take responsibility for the medical problems of their patients. Barton encouraged his colleagues to abandon the "cartoonist's" image of the psychiatrist sitting at the head of a "couch on which a wealthy neurotic woman reclines reciting trivia" in favor of a "new image of the psychiatrist [that] would stress ability as a well trained physician with technical knowledge and expertness required of a specialist."[28] Although psychoanalysts had once claimed that they were engaged in scientific examination of the patient's thought process, their method of sitting next to a couch appeared antiquated and not at all medical to the 1960s generation of researchers in academic psychiatry.[29]

As part of psychiatrists' discussions about how best to practice their specialty, researchers and psychoanalysts had significant conflicts around the most appropriate method of describing patients. In the 1950s and early 1960s, psychiatrists used case summaries in order to narrate both the patient history and experience with the treatment. Yet as treatments in the 1960s and 1970s increasingly involved administering medication and monitoring symptoms, some research-oriented psychiatrists began to complain that case summaries were too subjective and that patient reports were not sufficiently scientific. Instead, these researchers sought new ways of interacting with and representing patients, methods that decreased human variability in the interest of science.

The most active and vocal proponents of this approach toward patients were psychiatrist Robert Spitzer and researcher Jean Endicott of the New York State Psychiatric Institute. One of the hallmarks of Spitzer and Endicott's work was its emphasis on extracting information from patients in a way that could be replicated by multiple clinicians. Instead of presenting patients' stories, Spitzer and Endicott worked on symptom grouping, reliability between interviewers, and systematic diagnostic procedures.[30] Although he had been trained as a psychoanalyst, Spitzer was explicit that there was no room for the fuzziness that traditionally accompanied a psychoanalytic interaction with a patient: "Either the subject has made a statement which has substantially that meaning or the subject's verbal or overt behavior provides the evidence for the item. This term does not provide license to include inferences based on psychodynamic interpretations of motivation or of unconscious affect."[31] Although Spitzer sometimes acknowledged his own training, he worked hard to systematically eliminate psychoanalytic assumptions and approaches in his evaluation of patients and their symptoms.[32]

Spitzer and a number of others developed assessment tools that would ideally substitute for the usual clinical evaluation both for assessment of the patient and for determination of progress in medication and psychotherapy clinical trials. These assessment tools converted patient reports into symptoms that were in turn converted into numbers. Thus patients' progress through medication trials could be measured in rating scale values and manipulated with other patient statistics. Instead of comparing patients, researchers compared numbers, with the goal of reducing subjectivity in clinical trials. Spitzer and others hoped that these "objective" assessment tools would allow researchers to predict which patients would be likely to respond to medications. Not all assessment tools were the same—some investigators designed specific rating scales to use in specific circumstances. For example, a group at Brown University used the Kupfer Detre Scale (KDS-3A) to try to differentiate patients who might respond to lithium from those who might respond to tricyclic antidepressants.[33]

Psychoanalytically trained psychiatrists protested that rating scales assumed that patients were the same and that their response to medications would be the same. Instead, some argued that medications could have psycho-dynamic effects (such as the ways that patients' understood and expressed their feelings of hostility in the midst of depression).[34] Still, research psychiatrists by the late 1960s and 1970s increasingly insisted on the power of rating scales to compare populations of patients. Though psychoanalytically oriented psychiatrists published on the nature of depression, their interpretative framework was overshadowed by the quantitative methodology used by depression researchers.[35]

As researchers shifted their approach from patients' stories to quantitative analysis, patient symptoms became important primarily in groups. Allen Raskin, from the Psychopharmacology Research Branch at NIMH, evaluated a large number of patients across ten hospitals to determine the most important symptoms in depressed patients. In his study, the following factors seemed to be most important in depression: "1) depressed mood, 2) feelings of guilt and worthlessness, 3) hostility, 4) anxiety-tension, 5) cognitive loss and subjective uncertainty, 6) interest and involvement in activities, 7) somatic complaints, 8) sleep disturbance, 9) retardation in speech and behavior, 10) bizarre thoughts and behavior, 11) excitement and 12) denial of illness."[36] In determining that these factors were the most essential to describe depression, Raskin's group did not speculate on the effects of the demographics or personal experiences of his patient sample. Instead of looking at individuals and their contexts, many research groups by the 1970s employed statisticians to help them with increasingly complex data analysis.[37] In effect, researchers substituted the medication for the patient as the focus of the interaction, since the symptoms of clinical attention were highlighted by the medication interventions. The designers of the rating scales and symptom measurement exchanged one set of problems for another, though, as they reduced variability associated with individual clinician interviews but also reduced or eliminated much of the interviewer's opportunity to put patients' symptoms in context.

American psychiatrists were particularly eager to look for what appeared to be objective ways of defining depression as a disease, and medication response (as measured by rating scales) appeared abundantly objective. While British psychiatrists emphasized an older distinction between "endogenous" depression (arising from the patient) and "exogenous" or "reactive" depression (arising from the patient's response to his or her life circumstances), American psychiatrists complained that the terminology was too ambiguous to be used in clinical studies.[38] Further, the British breakdown of different types of depression did not match American researchers' experiences with medications. Washington University researcher Robert Woodruff emphasized in 1967 that the evidence for the endogenous-reactive split of depression was based on assumptión, not proven fact.[39] Without considering what was lost in converting patient stories to numbers, and without speculating on the role of life circumstances to symptoms, American psychiatrists embraced the opportunity to use quantitative measures in an effort to be more objective and more scientific.

By the 1970s, clinical trials of psychiatric treatments looked substantially different than the clinical trials only two decades earlier.[40] Psychiatric researchers were more likely to come from large academic medical centers such as Washington University in St. Louis or the New York State Psychiatric Institute. Further, researchers had become well versed in the language of science as applied to medicine in their study design and their biochemical explanations for drug effects.[41] Research studies increasingly used rating scales to quantify patient experiences with their medications, while researchers emphasized symptom tracking to measure improvement. This transformation in research methodology was exemplified by the NIMH Collaborative Depression Studies Program, a substantial, multicenter research group organized in the 1970s.[42]

The NIMH Collaborative Depression Studies Program involved a large-scale attempt to coordinate both basic science and clinical investigations on depression. The collaboration began with research psychiatrists' growing excitement about the results they were seeing with antidepressant medications. A number of investigators organized an NIMH conference on depression that defined the importance of work on the nosology, genetics, and pathophysiology of the illness. In 1979, the collaboration was formalized, and researchers began a naturalistic study of what were by this time commonly used treatments for depression.[43] As study coordinators and prominent psychiatrists Martin Katz and Gerald Klerman explained at the study's inception, conceptions of affective disorders had shifted a great deal over the previous several decades. Katz and Klerman said that the goal of the new NIMH collaboration was to "make possible the development of a coherent and valid psychobiologic theory of depression."[44] The clinical sites selected for inclusion in this collaboration included Massachusetts General/Harvard, Rush–Presbyterian–St. Luke's in Chicago, the University of Iowa, the New York State Psychiatric Institute, Washington University, and the NIMH. Two of these sites were also pivotal in defining the specific criteria for depression in the 1970s and 1980s. Researchers in this time period demonstrated their coherent vision of American psychiatry through their work on depression—that science could and should be the driving force in the field.

But at the same time that psychiatric researchers emphasized the science in their methodology, there were some research practices and assumptions that went unquestioned. Pharmaceutical companies began a practice of designing their own research studies and analyzing their own data.[45] Although it is difficult to assess the degree to which it influenced clinical trials by the 1970s and 1980s, it is clear that the pharmaceutical industry played a more active role in research by the time fluoxetine (Prozac) was introduced in the late 1980s. While the pharmaceutical industry collaborated with researchers and had some studies published in professional journals, critics have recently pointed out that industry research over the decades tended to bury negative results and to blur the boundaries between research and marketing.[46]

In addition, clinical trials on depressed patients more and more reinforced a circular definition of depression: depressed patients were those who could be shown to have responded to antidepressants, while antidepressants were medications that helped depressed patients.[47] Investigators worked hard to make sure that they had a reasonably homogenous subject population and freely excluded patients with schizophrenia-type diagnoses or substance abuse.[48] Further, some began to use medication response to divide patients into different groups by type of depression. This kind of typing of depression was also circular: patients were placed in categories based on their improvement with different types of medications, while psychiatrists claimed to be able to predict improvement with particular types of medication based on patients' depression type.[49]

Medication trials were not the only kinds of therapies that helped to define a specific diagnosis of depression, as new kinds of structured psychotherapies were developed in the 1970s and 1980s that functioned the same way.[50] The two main systems of psychotherapy that were used in research trials, often in combination with medication, were Cognitive Behavioral Therapy (CBT) and Interpersonal Psychotherapy (IPT). Aaron Beck and his colleagues at the University of Pennsylvania designed the highly structured CBT system in order to teach patients to counter the thought distortions that Beck argued were common in depression.[51] IPT, which was developed by Myrna Weissman and her colleagues primarily in a study population of depressed women, was based on trying to correct the interpersonal disruptions that Weissman found in her depressed subjects.[52] As Weissman explained in 1979, "the next decade will bring answers as to which type of psychotherapy to use with which drugs, for which depressed patient, and there will be a scientifically supportable rationale for the treatment of the different types of depression."[53] Thus specific psychotherapy, as well as specific medication, could be part of the scientific project of defining the disease of depression.

Defining Disease

In the first two decades of medication trials, there was no common agreed-upon method to make a diagnosis of depression. Depressive symptoms had appeared in the first edition of the *Diagnostic and Statistical Manual* (*DSM*), published by the APA in 1952, but only within disease groupings such as manic-depressive psychosis and neurotic reactions. In its attempt to reconcile the psychoanalysts' emphasis on conflict and reaction with the need to gather statistics on hospitalized mentally ill patients, the first *DSM* represented the state of flux that characterized psychiatry of the time.[54] Although the first edition of the *DSM* did not generate much enthusiasm within American psychiatry, it seemed adequate for most purposes through the end of the 1950s.[55] But in the 1960s the same research psychiatrists who had pushed for new assessment tools to evaluate patients began to move into the issue of psychiatric diagnosis. The main issue raised by the research psychiatrists was that it was extremely difficult to compare research studies without agreement on what was being studied. As a number of researchers pointed out, multiple psychiatrists seeing the same patient but coming to radically different conclusions about his or her diagnoses made the specialty appear unscientific.[56]

Robert Spitzer, who had worked on methodological innovation in psychiatric research with rating scales, also led the way to a reconceptualization of psychiatric diagnosis. Spitzer argued, in the context of the growing research enterprise of the 1960s and 1970s, that it was essential for psychiatrists across the country (and ideally around the world) to agree on how to assess and classify patients. For Spitzer and for others who were engaged in research activities, psychiatric diagnosis became a means of communication among professionals, not a statement about an individual patient's difficulty. With agreement as a focus, Spitzer made the explicit argument that a valid diagnosis (a diagnosis that reflected a disease in nature) mattered less than reliability (the agreement among professionals about the categories).[57] In other words, Spitzer said that it was less important to understand whether a mental problem was caused by a structural nerve problem, a biochemical abnormality, or conflicts within an individual's family (or other possible explanations)—it was more important that all psychiatrists agreed to describe the mental problem the same way. By substituting validity for reliability, Spitzer emphasized that psychiatric diagnostic classification did not depend on overcoming existing gaps in knowledge about the origins of mental disorders.[58]

As Spitzer and his colleagues increasingly focused on agreement among psychiatrists, they also became interested in ways in which technology (especially computers) could help reduce the fuzziness of the specialty. Psychiatrists and other researchers by the 1960s and 1970s hoped that computers could reduce or eliminate human bias in medicine.[59] In these decades, Spitzer and his New York State Psychiatric Institute collaborator Jean Endicott designed several computer simulations of diagnostic processes that revealed how difficult it was to establish consistent and reproducible psychiatric diagnoses.[60] In Spitzer and Endicott's voluminous publications, the closer the specialty came to adapting psychiatric assessment, data points, and diagnostic processes to computer algorithms, the closer psychiatry was to becoming a medical specialty based on objective, scientific research.

Not all psychiatrists agreed that computer applications signaled progress, however. Although APA medical director Walter Barton had been concerned that psychoanalytic interactions did not appear medical, he worried that the computer-systems approach eliminated necessary interpersonal qualities of the doctor-patient relationship: "There is encouragement to abandon the medical system approach in favor of the social system approach. Personal diagnosis may give way to the computer; the psychiatrist-psychotherapist may give way to the 'discount' therapist and to the friendly nonprofessional health visitor."[61] Further, the concept of specific diagnosis of any kind was not without detractors.[62] Psychiatrists agreed that they needed to improve their professional standing in a time of social and medical upheavals, but they differed somewhat about what strategies to take in this endeavor.[63] In the end, those who pushed for more diagnostic categories and greater reliability had more influence over the subsequent changes in the profession than those who emphasized psychiatry's doctor-patient relationships.

While researchers within the profession began to advocate for reliable diagnostic categories, the official diagnostic scheme of American psychiatry remained oriented around its original purpose of coding and record management, even for the second edition of the *DSM* that was published in 1968.[64] *DSM-II* did not explain methods for making diagnoses and was based on the assumption that psychiatrists would know particular mental diseases when they saw them. The volume itself was unimpressive—it was a cheaply produced, slim sheaf of papers held together with plastic fasteners and could be purchased from the APA Publications Office for $3.50 per copy (a library bound copy was available, but at extra cost).[65] Spitzer, who acted as a consultant for the last few years of the process of producing *DSM-II*, complained that *DSM-II* only tinkered with the categories from the first edition.[66] Indeed,

DSM-II was unable to be the kind of research resource that Spitzer wanted to support the advance of science in psychiatry since it did not define or really even describe specific mental diseases. Spitzer, with his colleagues in New York as well as a group of investigators at Washington University, worked to define specific categories of illnesses in what became the much more radical changes of *DSM-III*. On the way to *DSM-III*, Spitzer and other researchers for the first time named diagnostic criteria that would be used to consistently define mental illnesses, including depression.

In the 1970s, research groups at Washington University and the New York State Psychiatric Institute reviewed the growing mass of data on depression from medication trials and insisted that order needed to be brought into the research enterprise. In particular, it was essential that researchers have a common frame of reference in clinical trial patient selection that could be shared among research teams. The group at Washington University published a series of diagnostic symptoms in 1972 that became known as the Feighner criteria (named after the first author, John Feighner, who was a psychiatry resident at Washington University at that time). Feighner and his coauthors— Eli Robins, Samuel Guze, Robert Woodruff Jr., George Winokur, and Rodrigo Munoz—explained that there were five phases for establishing validity in psychiatric illness: clinical description, laboratory studies, establishment of the distinction from other disorders, follow-up studies on the original clinical descriptions, and family studies. The Feighner criteria included specific diagnostic instructions for a number of disorders, including primary affective disorders, schizophrenia, anxiety neurosis, obsessive-compulsive neurosis, phobic neurosis, hysteria, antisocial personality disorder, alcoholism, drug dependence, mental retardation, homosexuality, transsexualism, and anorexia nervosa. The authors explained that these disorders were chosen because there was some psychiatric literature that supported the validity of the diagnoses.[67]

But while this first effort to define psychiatric disease criteria highlighted validity, most of the subsequent diagnostic work emphasized reliability. As Spitzer's New York research group explained about their diagnostic scheme, the Research Diagnostic Criteria (RDC), in 1972, "In the absence of ultimate criteria for validating psychiatric diagnosis, such as are usually provided by various laboratory tests in other branches of medicine, we are thrown back on determining its reliability, since the degree of agreement between diagnosticians necessarily represents the upper limit of validity."[68] As psychiatrists focused more and more on reliability, depression became the test case on which the research groups in St. Louis and New York hammered out consensus.

Depression was one of the specific diagnoses within the 1972 Feighner criteria but was significantly expanded in Spitzer's RDC, research criteria originally developed for the NIMH Collaborative Depression Studies Program. While the Feighner criteria had described only depression, mania, and secondary depression as primary affective disorders, the RDC separated depressive and bipolar disorders and included eleven subtypes of depressive disorders: primary, secondary, recurrent unipolar, psychotic, incapacitating, endogenous, agitated, retarded, situational, simple, and predominant mood. The RDC also included minor depressive disorder, intermittent depressive disorder, and cyclothymic personality.[69] The RDC for depression required a symptom of depressed mood, plus an additional set of symptoms and a minimum time frame of one month. The RDC also insisted that patients needed either to have sought help for their condition or to have been noticed by others to need help.[70]

While Spitzer played a key role in helping to design research criteria for disease, this position did not translate into major power within the APA. At the time when Spitzer and others were quietly building the basis for a revolution in psychiatric diagnosis, leaders within the APA were focused on responding to national political challenges and social and cultural upheavals.[71] The APA was also attempting to define psychiatry against an increasingly active and vocal American Psychological Association (APsychA), which was questioning the difference between psychological therapies and psychiatric practice.[72] In this context, the radical nature of Spitzer's work in evolving the *DSM-III* only became apparent to leaders within psychiatry and psychology as the research criteria were increasingly formalized into diagnostic instructions.

While the Feighner criteria and the RDC were widely used in research settings, they generally did not inform the practice of the rank and file of American psychiatrists. Spitzer and his colleagues in a variety of medical centers in the 1970s began to educate more clinically oriented psychiatrists (beyond just researchers) about the need for criteria in psychiatric diagnosis. Further, Spitzer and others began the challenging process of writing, defending, and moving the third edition of the *DSM* through administrative and bureaucratic channels. As Spitzer described at the time and in reflection, *DSM-III* represented a major change for psychiatrists. Its design and approval processes were long and difficult, particularly because many within psychiatry were caught by surprise by the magnitude of the change. Spitzer had to contend with critics who were involved early and those who appeared on the scene late in the game. He also had the political difficulties of explaining and justifying certain aspects of the new diagnostic scheme that appeared to be offensive to representatives of the APsychA and to psychoanalysts within the profession who believed that they were being left out.[73] Further, Spitzer faced a significant number of psychiatrists who complained that *DSM-III* represented a major loss to psychiatry by eliminating a psychodynamic view of the patient.[74]

As *DSM-III* was being developed, depression came to occupy an increasingly important and distinct place in psychiatric nomenclature, as this criteria-based diagnosis appeared to exemplify the new model for psychiatric illness. But it also illustrated the limitations of developing diagnostic definitions through consensus. Researchers had looked at populations of patients who were in the hospital with what was commonly understood to be depression based on response to medication. Patients' symptoms were then counted and analyzed to see which best characterized the population of patients. Further, as with medication trials, patients with alcoholism or drug dependence were not included in evolving discussions around diagnosis of depression. The RDC had named possible subtypes of depression, but researchers argued about these subtypes, what caused them, and how they might respond to different medications. For the new classification system, etiology was set aside in favor of description of symptoms. It did not matter why or how patients developed symptoms, just as long as researchers could all agree on the significance of those symptoms.

In order to get from the more narrow focus of the RDC to the general purpose *DSM-III* criteria, Spitzer worked with a group of psychiatrists who had been doing research on depression to come up with what he identified as a consensus diagnosis.[75] Spitzer sent out written case descriptions of patients and had members of his group make comments and suggestions for how the cases fit with the working criteria. The work group, which included well-respected researchers and academic psychiatrists Donald Klein, Rachel Gittelman, Kenneth Solomon, Michael Sheehy, Edward Sacher, and Arthur Rifkin, had the opportunity to voice significant complaints and make substantive comments about the proposed criteria for *DSM-III*. It was also clear that Spitzer and a number of his group were concerned about separating their diagnostic definition of depression from the ideas of the psychoanalysts. But though Spitzer said that he was working with a consensus from a work group, he tightly contained the discussion around the diagnosis to move on with the production of *DSM-III*. At several points, Spitzer sent out questionnaires to his group to ask their opinions about the criteria. In these questionnaires, the responders had a series of complete questions but had room for only a check mark to indicate whether they agreed with that point.[76]

In the discussion over the diagnostic criteria for depression to be included in *DSM-III*, the group working with Spitzer repeatedly raised the issue of different types of depression that responded differently to treatment. A few American psychiatrists advocated adoption of the British distinction between endogenous (presumably arising through an internal process) and exogenous (or reactive to external events) depression. Spitzer, however, wanted to avoid specific types of depression in his criteria in order to make the overall category of depression quite broad and to maximize agreement among psychiatrists. As he explained in a cover letter to a work-group questionnaire, "The criteria in *DSM-III* were not intended to limit the diagnosis of a depressive syndrome to patients with endogenous phenomenology. Studies have found that the depressive episodes of bipolar as well as recurrent unipolar patients may have few endogenous features and that even psychotic or incapacitated patients may also fail to have sufficient endogenous features to qualify for an 'endogenous' syndrome." Spitzer commented that the criteria were supposed to be tight enough to not diagnose "every 'slump' as a full depressive syndrome" but loose enough to get people back into treatment after relapse.[77] Further, the treatment categories needed to deal with loosely defined subtypes of depression that had been discussed in the previous decade. As researcher Gerald Klerman and his coauthors, including Spitzer, argued in 1979, diagnoses such as "neurotic depression" remained problematic because of major disagreements about what this term meant.[78] Instead, Spitzer and others advocated for putting all kinds of depression together in one category with the hope that research in the future with this category would help to uncover causes for the illness.

Although Spitzer worked hard to achieve consensus within the group of people working on the *DSM-III* category of depression, there was no unanimity within the field. Bernard Carroll, the developer of the Dexamethasone Suppression Test (DST) (see below), objected to Spitzer's efforts to lump together all types of depression within one category.[79] University of Iowa researcher Nancy Andreasen, who later joined Spitzer's depression work group, published an article in 1979 complaining that "because periods of sadness or grief are ubiquitous in human experience and because sadness is often accompanied by such typical depressive symptoms as sleeplessness or loss of interest, the concept of depression can be overinclusive and heterogeneous."[80] Clearly, there were still significant differences among the researchers on types of depression, core clinical symptoms, and relationship to outcome. But despite some dissenting opinions, a few unpleasant letters, and publications that suggested that the category did not capture the complexity of depressive illness, Spitzer and his group finalized the criteria for major depression in time for the 1980 production of *DSM-III*.

In the end, the *DSM-III* criteria for depression were similar to those of the RDC, but a few differences illustrated the shift in purpose from the RDC to *DSM-III*. First, the *DSM-III* criteria were more easily met by a larger portion of the population. The RDC for depression required dysphoric mood, as well as five of seven symptoms (appetite and sleep had to be decreased). Further, the symptoms had to be present for at least a month. In the new *DSM-III* criteria, though, dysphoric mood was still required, but only four of eight symptoms needed to be present, and appetite and sleep could be either increased or decreased. In addition, the symptoms only needed to be present for two weeks. While the RDC criteria had been designed to ensure a homogenous patient population for research trials, the *DSM-III* criteria were intended to make sure that patients could get into treatment. Thus the bar to diagnosis was lower in the new diagnostic manual.[81] The other way in which the *DSM-III* criteria were different from the RDC and other research measures was in the focus of the diagnosis. While the mood descriptors for both the RDC and *DSM-III* definitions included "depressed, sad, blue, hopeless, low, down in the dumps, irritable," the RDC mood descriptors also included "despondent, fearful, worried, or discouraged."[82] The new criteria allowed for shorter episodes before diagnosing patients, but excluded experiences that might be confused with anxiety (which had its own set of diagnostic criteria).

DSM-III represented a major change for psychiatric theory and prac-tice, particularly with regard to depression. For the first time, psychiatrists outside research settings were being instructed on how to make diagnoses using specific criteria. The architects of *DSM-III* were well aware that the new manual represented a significant departure from usual psychiatric practice, and they offered training sessions within the APA in order to facilitate clinician use of the manual.[83] Spitzer and others stressed the importance of having all psychiatrists across the country (and even the world) speak the same language about depression. As researchers and clinicians published in the psychiatric literature through the 1970s and 1980s, their discussion of depression increas-ingly focused on specific criteria that described a specific category, treated with a specific medication.

The 1980 publication of *DSM-III* was by no means the end of the conver-sation about diagnosis for Spitzer and the others who worked on the new diagnostic manual. Still, even while controversy remained about how to handle the many problems that were discussed around *DSM-III*, a major change had occurred within psychiatry, one that could not be easily overlooked or dismissed. After *DSM-III*, diagnosis was explicitly made by assessing for the presence and absence of psychiatric symptoms in patients. Within *DSM-III*, the disease category of major depressive disorder appeared for the first time and was formally described. Further, although some psychiatrists complained about symptom checklists, they did not generally point fingers at depression's status as a diagnostic category defined by specific symptoms. Indeed, the diagnosis of depression appeared to represent success in the completion of *DSM-III*.

Although the 1980 publication of *DSM-III* had a tremendous effect on psychiatry over a relatively short period of time, particularly in the area of depression, Spitzer and others involved in the diagnostic process were not content to leave the manual alone. After a conference to evaluate *DSM-III* in October 1983, Spitzer and work groups based around different diagnostic categories were asked to evaluate those categories and propose changes. As with his work groups for *DSM-III*, Spitzer tightly contained the discussions around the proposed changes in the criteria after researchers made their presentations in the 1983 conference. Indeed, a few changes in the criteria for major depressive disorder appear to have been made by Spitzer and then presented to the group for ratification. While members of the work group were asked whether they wanted to retain a melancholic subtype of depression, they were apparently not asked whether it was appropriate to eliminate some mood descriptors from the core features of the illness. Without comment, irritability disappeared as a descriptor for mood in major depressive disorder.[84]

In 1987, a new revised edition of the *DSM* was published, *DSM-IIIR*. In the revised criteria for depression, there was no longer a requirement that depressed mood be present along with other criteria. Instead, the patient needed to meet five of nine possible criteria, although the diagnosis required either depressed mood or loss of interest or pleasure. In addition, the number of mood descriptors was significantly reduced, and irritability was no longer mentioned in adults (although it was specifically mentioned for children). Other symptoms included appetite or weight disturbance, sleep disturbance, psychomotor agitation or retardation, fatigue or loss of energy, feelings of worthlessness or guilt, decreased concentration, and recurrent thoughts of death. A subtype of depression, identified as "Melancholic Type," included nine criteria and specified that the patient needed to meet five of them. One of the criteria introduced for *DSM-IIIR* was response to "specific and adequate somatic antidepressant therapy."[85]

While some inside and outside the profession had criticized the concept and/or the execution of *DSM-III*, by the time of *DSM-IIIR* the controversy had begun to fade as categorical diagnoses seemed to be fairly well entrenched.[86]

Further, there was little if any criticism of the fact that depression was now a major category of illness. Indeed, the specific category of depression that was used on a research basis in the 1970s and then codified in 1980 became even more important in the 1980s. Even though major depressive disorder was only one of the 227 diagnoses within *DSM-III* and one of 253 diagnoses within *DSM-IIIR,* by the 1980s depression appeared to be a grave, growing, and often undiagnosed public health concern.

Medications to Molecules

At the same time that Robert Spitzer and others were beginning to define a new classification system for psychiatric disease, researchers increasingly applied information about medication effects to create molecular models for depression. Although clinicians and researchers did not have a clear idea about the precise nature of depression, many researchers fell back on what they did know: that psychiatric medications worked. While psychiatric medications were originally given because their effects seemed to oppose the clinical presentation of the patients (that is, medications that would cause euphoria were given to counter depressive symptoms), researchers by the 1960s began to take this reasoning farther to make inferences about what was happening in patients' brains before and with treatment based on observed effects of medication. In animal experiments, researchers found that so-called antidepressant medications had effects on two recently discovered neurotransmitters: serotonin and norepinephrine. Psychiatrists inferred that since medications that increased the levels of these neurotransmitters caused euphoria in animals, depression must be caused by a deficiency in these neurotransmitters in the human nervous system.

Both clinicians and researchers were easily able to translate the idea of treating symptoms with their opposite into medication effects with the new language of neurotransmitters. For example, private practitioner T. R. Robie explained that iproniazid worked in depression by protecting serotonin in the brain: "Serotonin, allowed free activity in the brain, is perhaps the most energetic releaser of reserve power in the human machine, and this effect will overcome melancholia in a majority of cases within 2 to 4 weeks."[87] Joseph Schildkraut, a major researcher in brain physiology, explained this in basic science terms in his often-cited 1965 review on the theory of depression, which he called the "catecholamine hypothesis." Schildkraut emphasized that drugs that decrease norepinephrine cause sedation or depression in animals, while drugs that increase norepinephrine, including MAOIs and amphetamine, "are associated with behavioral stimulation or excitement and generally exert an antidepressant effect in man."[88] While Schildkraut cautioned that this theory could not account for all medication effects or all forms of depression, his hypothesis became (and continues to be) a major working theory for depression.[89] Although Schildkraut's hypothesis was much more technical than Robie's explanation, both reasoned backward about the cause of depression from the effects of medication that seemed to work on depressive states, states that were themselves defined by medication effect.[90]

But though the catecholamine hypothesis was attractive, it still could not organize all discussions around depression in the 1970s because the animal model did not have direct human applications. Further, researchers by this time had not succeeded in achieving agreement around terminology. In 1975, Anthony D'Agostino, a psychiatrist at the Loyola University Stritch School of Medicine, commented, "Unfortunately, in the mid-1970s we are still unable to agree on whether depression is a disease, a scapegoat phenomenon, a problem in living, a conditioned response to a series of more or less accidental environmental contingencies, an overly insightful existential awareness of the futility of man's struggle against the inevitability of death, or all of the above."[91] But research psychiatrists in the 1970s did make particular efforts to synthesize all the theories about depression in order to emphasize its nature as a real disease. For example, in 1974 New York State Psychiatric Institute researcher Donald Klein made complex charts and graphs describing signs, symptoms, and etiologies of depression. In 1975, depression researcher Hagop Akiskal engaged in a Herculean effort to synthesize ten widely divergent ideas about how patients got to be depressed.[92] Yet research psychiatrists' ultimate goal was to find a biological sign—preferably a laboratory test—that could definitively define depression.

In order to find some kind of objective measure that could be administered to patients to evaluate their level of depression and their response to medication, some researchers tracked the level of MHPG, a metabolite of norepinephrine, in patients' urine. Psychiatrists reasoned that if norepinephrine was low in depression, MHPG levels would also be low. It was obviously impossible to check norepinephrine or MHPG levels in the brain, but the levels in urine might make a reasonable approximation. This was a promising theory, as psychiatrists searched for some kind of marker for depression that they could use to screen cases and measure objective improvement. But MHPG levels, while significant in some studies, did not turn out to have the predictive power that researchers originally hoped.[93] Researchers expressed enthusiasm about other markers as well, including 5-HIAA (a serotonin metabolite), and found some significance in small studies, but they never found enough consistent evidence of biological markers to allow for a broad-scale biological test for depression.[94] Other researchers used platelet level of monoamine oxidase (MAO), an enzyme in the neurotransmitter pathway thought to have something to do with depression, as an approximation of brain MAO activity to see if levels predicted depression. But since MAO levels were tied to a specific antidepressant—MAOIs—this biological marker was less useful for depression in general.[95]

One of the most promising biological tests in the late 1970s and early 1980s was the DST. Developed in part by University of Michigan psychiatrist Bernard Carroll, the DST took advantage of increased medical interest in stress hormones, particularly cortisol.[96] Researchers speculated that depression was linked to increased stress hormones. When dexamethasone, an artificial stress hormone, was administered to a normal subject, it would decrease, or suppress, endogenous stress hormones. For depressed patients, however, the stress hormones could not be suppressed, and cortisol levels would remain elevated.[97] Researchers were enthusiastic about the possibilities of the DST, and wrote optimistically about it even when their study results showed positive DST results in fewer than 50 percent of depressed patients.[98] Although the DST never entirely disappeared, its clinical utility did not become as broad as originally anticipated. As one group that tested the DST, along with other biochemical markers, explained in 1981, "An underlying promise in the elucidation of neuroendocrine function in patients is that a neuroendocrine abnormality will be a reflection of a more primary neurotransmitter abnormality."[99] Researchers passionately hoped that their work in depression would uncover some kind of biological marker for depression that would allow them to be part of the technological revolution in medicine.[100]

Another set of tools that appeared promising were those associated with the newly (re)formed field of genetics, as psychiatrists attempted to find a familial form of depression.[101] In 1979, George Winokur of the University of Iowa described "pure depressive disease" (that is, without mania or alcoholism) and looked at the patients with this form of the illness and their families. Winokur suggested that the familial cases, those with a positive family history of pure depressive disease, and the sporadic cases were actually different types of illness with different responses to treatment.[102] He followed up this study with another one that differentiated pure depressive disease from a group of ailments he identified as "depression-spectrum" disorders, which included family history of alcoholism or antisocial personality.[103] For Winokur and other genetic researchers, the question was not whether depression was a biologically based (and therefore heritable) illness—they assumed it was. The question instead was how it was transmitted through the generations.

Not all of the psychiatric research enterprise was fully committed to a biological, laboratory-based approach, though. Psychoanalysts Silvano Arieti and Jules Bemporad pointed out in 1980 that psychological theories could not be ignored: "Although appreciative of the contribution of biochemical hypotheses to the etiology of depression and the efficacy of organic treatments on some aspects of the depressive syndrome, we hold the view that psychological mechanisms, which have recently suffered neglect, remain important to the understanding and treatment of affective disorders."[104] Though Arieti and Bemporad attempted to demonstrate that it was possible to do research with psychoanalytic data, most psychiatrists could not bridge the gap between psychoanalysts' focus on the individual and researchers' focus on numbers in either laboratory values or statistical measure of patient symptoms.

Researchers' work with laboratory studies and genetic investigations, along with the specific *DSM-III* diagnostic category of depression, reinforced the idea that depression was a disease of the brain. As the psychiatric leaders within the APA and academic departments increasingly became oriented toward biological approaches, the treatment of depression and its diagnostic specificity appeared to be at the forefront of the new modern psychiatry.[105] But depression not only helped psychiatrists reimagine their specialty in terms of its similarity to general medicine in laboratory applications and science. In addition, depression offered an opportunity for psychiatrists to promote the disease (and their expertise in treating it) to larger and larger segments of the American population.

Expansion

By the 1980s, depression appeared to be a growing problem. But it was growing at least in part because researchers began to advocate intervention into patients' lives beyond episodes of acute depression. For example, a surge of interest in lithium led a number of investigators to explore whether lithium could help patients with manic-depression during their depressive episodes, or even help those with only depression. Those who focused on lithium tended to try to treat patients during their periods of wellness rather than just during their periods of depression.[106] Further, as psychiatrists expanded the scope of the depression diagnosis, the pool of potential patients appeared to include the entire nation. Instead of just focusing on patients already in treatment, academic psychiatrists began to explore the community as a whole to try to identify people who were not previously diagnosed.

Depression research helped foster new collaborations between psychiatrists and epidemiologists.[107] As psychiatric researchers and clinicians emphasized depression's importance in the community, they increasingly worked with epidemiologists to explore depression populations on the model of chronic diseases such as heart disease. Psychiatrists explained that depression became chronic when patients still had symptoms after treatment or later relapses. Further, as with other chronic diseases, community surveillance might yield not only undiagnosed cases but also undiscovered risk factors.[108] Psychiatrists who invoked the language of depression as a chronic disease did so in order to emphasize the severity of the illness and its impact on the nation. Thus, with the combination of psychiatry and epidemiology, depression was both a psychiatric illness and a public health problem.[109]

With the criteria provided by the RDC and *DSM-III*, researchers began to examine diagnostic patterns in a variety of patient populations. Although there had been several large-scale epidemiological studies of mental illness in the 1960s and 1970s, research psychiatrists complained that the clinical interviews in the older studies were incomplete and difficult to compare.[110] Further, the differences in data collection and diagnostic assessment had rendered comparisons of rates of mental illness between different countries virtually impossible.[111] The Epidemiological Catchment Area (ECA) study was the first large-scale epidemiological study performed after the specific diagnostic criteria of *DSM-III* in the early 1980s. In the ECA study, researchers used *DSM-III* criteria to screen the general population to estimate the prevalence of psychiatric disease and found enormous reservoirs of untreated psychiatric illness in the United States.[112]

Psychiatrists used epidemiological studies such as the ECA to make pleas for more resources and attention toward the national problem of undiagnosed and untreated depression. Further, psychiatrists increasingly made the argument that depression was so common and affected such a variety of individuals that primary care physicians needed to be educated to recognize and treat it.[113] Psychiatric researchers began to adapt depression rating scales in order to design screening tools to address the major problems of morbidity and even suicide among those with undiagnosed depression in primary care settings.[114] Psychiatrists emphasized that depression could be dangerous if uncovered, but they also stressed its ease of treatment. As psychiatrist Sidney Zisook explained in *Postgraduate Medicine* in 1980, "Depression is a common malady that can cause mild complaints or great suffering and, in its extreme form, can be life threatening. With careful diagnosis and appropriate choice of medication, dramatic response to drug treatment is possible."[115] With the ongoing use of screening tools and diagnostic instruments, primary care practitioners were introduced to the idea that they, too, could have the satisfaction of diagnosing depression and watching their patients recover. Although the introduction of easy-to-use medications such as Prozac certainly helped spread enthusiasm for treating depression among primary care physicians, psychiatrists began to educate primary care providers about depression a decade before these medications were widely available.

The NIMH Collaborative Depression Studies Program—which was still going on in the early 1980s—also helped to raise awareness about the primary care treatment of depression. The initial study was intended to track patients through their treatment, but investigators became concerned that patients in the observation part of the study were not being adequately treated even before their referral to the study. As study lead Martin Keller explained in 1982, the investigators expected to find that study patients—those who had been diagnosed with and treated for depression prior to enrollment in the study—would already have experienced significant treatments for depression; yet in fact many of the patients had not had a trial of any medication at all, and a significant number had been undertreated by the standards of the investigators.[116] This finding raised the alarm about primary care physicians in particular, and a series of studies ensued that purported to demonstrate that most cases of depression were undetected by internists and general practitioners.[117] With these findings and their increased enthusiasm and concern for depression, Keller and his group led a campaign to educate family practice physicians about the importance of diagnosing and treating depression.[118]

At the same time that psychiatrists worked with epidemiologists and primary care physicians to identify the population extent of depression, they also continued to expand the number of individuals who could be diagnosed with depression by broadening the symptom criteria. For example, psychiatrists increasingly used the concept of chronic dysthymia (or chronic low-grade depression), a diagnosis similar to depression but requiring fewer symptoms. But not only did dysthymia potentially describe larger numbers of patients (more people would meet the low threshold for diagnosis), psychiatrists also expressed concern about a phenomenon they called "double depression," or a major depressive episode on top of chronic dysthymia.[119] Researchers, intent on spreading the word about depression treatments, emphasized that there were portions of the population who were experiencing symptoms but were not benefiting from the scientific revolution within psychiatry.

Throughout their discussions of depression in both medical and popular literatures, psychiatrists emphasized the need to educate the public about the nature of depression as a disease, its core symptoms, and its treatment. Professionals worried that the public did not know that depressive symptoms constituted a disease, and they stressed again and again the need to uncover cases of depression with the clear implication that patients could not or would not diagnose themselves. Further, psychiatrists argued that even those who knew that depression was a disease needed further education because they might unknowingly stop their treatment once they felt better. Instead, researchers suggested that depression was a chronic disease, one that required maintenance treatment rather than just treatment of acute episodes.[120] Thus many research studies on depressed patients led directly to public education campaigns to enlighten the public about depression and existing patients about the need to continue treatment.

The NIMH Collaborative Depression Studies Program took up concerns about the management of chronic depression. In one of the study's initial papers, the authors worried that recovery for patients was more prolonged than originally expected.[121] Further, even after a year, a quarter of the patients still had not recovered from the initial episode, and a significant number had relapsed despite treatment.[122] As the NIMH study continued, researchers highlighted the problems of patients with three or more episodes of depression and suggested that these patients were at the highest risk for future relapse and should be continued in treatment.[123] In 1985, the group published consensus guidelines that reported that 50 to 85 percent of patients with an episode of depression would suffer another episode. Further, the authors articulated the need for greater education: "Because the preventive treatment of recurrent mood disorders is clearly effective for large numbers of persons suffering from these conditions, and because a substantial proportion does not now seek treatment or are not accurately diagnosed, systematic efforts should be made to bring about a greater awareness of and understanding by both health professionals and the public of the nature and effective treatment of these illnesses."[124] NIMH researchers hypothesized that previously undiagnosed individuals in the general population would come forward and seek treatment once they understood their symptoms. The Collaborative Depression Studies Program's suggestions translated into public education with NIMH's Depression Awareness, Recognition, and Treatment campaign in the late 1980s, a public health effort designed to educate the public about depression and get people into appropriate treatment.[125]

Psychiatric researchers' interest in the widespread extent and subtle forms of depression illustrated their shift in thinking about depression as a disease. As Myrna Weissman, the prolific Yale researcher, remarked in 1976, classifying depression as a chronic disease had significant public health consequences: "Current health policy in the United States is focused on chronic diseases with high mortality. Mental disorders that have a high morbidity and potential mortality, such as depression, also require long-range comprehensive planning."[126] Psychiatrists' shift toward investigating the long-term, chronic aspects of depression changed the focus of their research and allowed them to expand their professional scope both by extending the time course of the necessary intervention (acute episodes as well as longer-term maintenance) and their patient population (those already in treatment as well as those untreated). In addition, by explaining that depression was a chronic disease of enormous magnitude, psychiatric researchers made explicit claims about the need to improve funding and national attention toward depression.[127] In their quest to define a reliable diagnosis of depression, researchers and epidemiologists expanded the reach of American psychiatry.

In 1986, Emory psychiatrist Alan Stoudemire and colleagues from other academic sites estimated the economic burden of depression in the United States. By assuming, based on epidemiological data, that 1 to 3 percent of the population might be depressed at one time and that 60 percent of suicides were due to depression, Stoudemire and his colleagues calculated the cost of productivity loss with depression and suicide, hospitalization, outpatient care, and medications. They concluded that depression cost approximately $16 billion a year in both direct and indirect costs.[128] These calculations illustrated in stark terms the tremendous burden of depression and its care in the country—but they also illustrated how important depression had become to American psychiatry. At the beginning of the twentieth century, psychiatrists were concerned about the costs of care and the national implications of mental illness, but they did not have a disease model of depression as it appeared by the 1990s. Stoudemire's 1986 calculation was based on specific diagnostic criteria, epidemiological data, and an infrastructure of treatment—all of which had become key to psychiatrists' self-definition.

Stoudemire's assumptions about depression's extent and costs to society reflect the American context in which depression emerged as a disease. Although contemporary psychiatrists emphasize the global burden of depression, the ways in which depression was defined and conceptualized illustrate contingencies in its evolution in American society and psychiatry. While Americans were preoccupied with anxiety at the middle of the twentieth century, depression emerged in the second half of the century and became one of the most discussed and studied diseases in psychiatric literature. Further, diagnostic criteria were a particular American invention, especially the assumption that identification of symptoms out of social and cultural context represents an appropriate way to make a diagnosis.

Although neuroses (and later anxiety) were important concepts within American psychiatry and society up through midcentury, depression played a more significant role than anxiety in the reconstruction of the profession in the second half of the century. David Healy has argued that Americans' scare over the addictive properties of anti-anxiety medications (such as Miltown) in the 1950s and 1960s led to abandonment of this form of treatment (and presumably professional caution about anxiety in general).[129] Yet it may also be that research psychiatrists, eager to distance themselves from the psychoanalytic portion of the profession, avoided anxiety because it was too close to neurosis. That certainly appeared to be the perception of researchers such as Robert Spitzer, who tried to have neurosis removed from psychiatric nomenclature.[130] Since much of the redefinition of depression as a set of symptoms (rather than conflicts) took place as part of a move away from psychoanalytic theories, maybe it is not a surprise that anxiety (as tied to neuroses) did not have the same appeal as depression for later twentieth-century researchers.[131]

Not only did American researchers have their own relationship to neuroses, but also they conceptualized psychiatric disease classification in a uniquely American way. Psychiatrist John Feighner, who got his research start as the first author on the 1972 diagnostic criteria that bore his name, reflected in 1979 on the importance of nosology for American psychiatry. Feighner pointed out that nosology helped clinicians by assisting them in predicting treatment response, and helped researchers by ensuring homogenous groups for comparison. He contrasted the existential French diagnostic approach with the "more pragmatic, data-oriented American nosological process."[132] Not only was the new nosology American and intensely practical, but also it had the virtue of making psychiatry appear more scientific within the increasingly technical nature of late-twentieth-century medical practice.[133] As *DSM-III* Advisory Committee member Paul Chodoff remarked in 1986, the point of view of *DSM-III*, "a more objective and less theory-bound way of looking at disturbed behavior—has augmented a general trend toward the medicalization of the phenomena of psychiatry."[134] Feighner and Chodoff echoed many of the arguments that Spitzer had made over the decades about the importance of being able to gather data in a systematic way and to manipulate that data to allow for future discovery. By many accounts, the changes wrought in American psychiatry by the emergence of *DSM-III* made it a more scientific specialty.

But American faith in science has obscured some of the problems with the diagnosis of depression.[135] Psychiatrists assumed that symptoms were more valuable than stories to compare patients and their treatments. But while the use of symptoms and scale measurements can appear objective, it is still impossible to control or to predict how or why patients endorse symptoms the way they do.[136] Further, the elimination of patients' stories seems to have had the consequence of treating all symptoms as equivalent. Although someone who meets *DSM* criteria for depression because of a relationship breakup might need a different approach from someone who meets *DSM* criteria without any apparent precipitant, the model of treating (with medication) based on a symptom checklist suggests that a computer (or a magazine questionnaire) could function as well as a psychiatrist to diagnose mental illness.

Not only have modern psychiatrists de-emphasized the value of human interactions in their reduction of stories to statistical data, but also they expanded the ways in which people can meet criteria for mental illness. Throughout the second half of the century, more and more researchers added more and more features—and consequently potential and actual patients—to the group of depressed patients. In the shift of the diagnostic criteria in the Feighner, RDC, and *DSM* symptom lists, fewer symptoms were required for shorter periods of time as the diagnosis was revised. Further, the vague noncontextual questions about mood symptoms used in epidemiological surveys cast a broad net to search for possible cases of depression. At no time did researchers call a halt to this process of expanding territory in depression—depression researchers could definitely agree on the national problem of depression, and no prevalence estimates seemed too large.

The process of moving from a reliable to a valid diagnosis of depression appears to have stalled. Although Robert Spitzer and the others involved in making new diagnostic categories emphasized that symptom-based criteria and checklists were only the beginning of the process of defining mental disease, existing diagnostic categories have achieved the status of scientifically proven truth. Researchers are experimenting with shorter and shorter screening instruments for depression, but there is no apparent plan to change the current diagnostic procedure.[137] Although there has been active discussion about adopting a different approach toward personality disorders, the current plans for *DSM-V* suggest that depression will continue to be diagnosed via a constellation of symptoms.[138]

Researchers' initial decisions to put aside questions of etiology in the diagnosis may have resulted in driving underground assumptions about the origins of depression. David Faust of Brown and University of Minnesota researcher Richard Miner complained in 1986 about the "statistical definition of normality and abnormality" and that the *DSM* criteria did in fact include theory about mental disease buried within the symptom-based categories.[139] There *is* an assumption within the *DSM* criteria of depression—that these symptoms are due to a disease process rather than a normal response to a stress. The clear intention of the disease category is to provide clinicians with guidelines for when to treat patients to remove the symptoms. This is not an atheoretical process.[140]

Although researchers have obscured some of the ways in which the diagnosis of depression was constructed, it is obvious that the discussions about depression have increasingly taken place outside medical and research settings. Yet there has been little public outcry against the more and more energetic psychiatrist assertions about the widespread nature of depression. Critics of psychiatry have blasted the profession (and the pharmaceutical industry) for promoting psychiatric illness onto what they claim is a gullible public.[141] But the American public has not been a passive recipient of psychiatric treatment. Instead, many Americans have embraced the idea of depression within a system of sophisticated, informed consumerism.

Chapter 3

American Moods and the Consumer Solution

In 1963, *Business Week* reported that "a new kind of pep pill is going through clinical tests at selected clinics and mental hospitals all around the country. But it didn't start out as a pep pill—or, to be less colloquial, a psychic energizer. Abbott Laboratories of Chicago developed it originally as a drug to lower blood pressure." The author enthusiastically projected that this pill would have a huge market since one to two out of five patients routinely went to their doctors without specific complaints—those patients might be depressed, and they might respond to the new medication. The author speculated that the pill could give a life to people who were grieving or stressed, and it had the advantage of being readily available to the "ordinary physician," who could treat patients quickly instead of sending them for more prolonged psychiatric care.[1]

This *Business Week* forecast of the potential market for a "pep pill" was right, despite the fact that at the time this article was written, depression as a specific illness did not exist. The criteria that would eventually comprise major depressive disorder were a decade away from their first formulation. Psychiatrists had barely started doing medication trials on hospitalized patients. Yet the *Business Week* author could see tremendous potential in the idea of a pill to improve "pep." Medications for mental ailments such as anxiety had already had a strong impact on the growing market for pharmaceuticals in the United States by the late 1950s and early 1960s.[2] In subsequent decades, medications for depression also became big news. But depression's expanding appeal within popular literature did not just tap into American enthusiasm about medications. Instead, depression treatment by the 1970s and 1980s fit Americans' growing preoccupation with self-improvement, the availability of methods by which to change the self with consumption, as well as ongoing social and political crises and individual and national mood.

Recent critics of the pharmaceutical industry have complained that direct-to-consumer (DTC) advertising in the late 1990s manufactured desire for antidepressant medications by convincing individuals that their lives needed improvement through chemistry.[3] But the consumer desire for remedies for depression existed decades before the advent of DTC marketing. The reason that recent advertising has been so successful is that the market for external methods to lift mood already existed. By the time that advertisements for products such as Prozac appeared in magazines, Americans had already been sold on the importance and prevalence of depression as a disease and its particular importance to the United States. Further, Americans were already convinced that individual happiness was an essential part of life—a pill (or other purchasable commodity) could be the answer to life's problems.[4]

At the same time that psychiatrists were observing the effects of medications on mood states, formalizing a diagnosis of depression, and speculating on the role of brain chemicals, American readers of popular magazines were engaged in related discussions about recognizing and treating depression and the role of the disease in American consumer culture.[5] While physicians were definitely part of these popular discussions, commentators felt free to elaborate on—and even criticize—psychiatrist contributions to magazine literature. Psychiatric researchers engaged in large-scale clinical trials had argued that the public needed better education about depression so that undetected cases of the illness could be diagnosed and treated. Yet as psychiatrist Peter Kramer found with his 1993 best seller *Listening to Prozac*, the immediate enormous sales of and popular enthusiasm for fluoxetine (Prozac) shortly after its introduction in the late 1980s suggested that millions of Americans did not need much convincing that depression treatment would help them.[6]

Depression—as a mood descriptor instead of an economic condition—appeared in popular magazines for the first time in the mid-1950s with a grumpy piece by E. B. White, the *New Yorker* contributor and well-known author of *Stuart Little*, on the emotional consequences of holiday shopping.[7] Popular press articles about depression began in earnest in the 1960s with a number of conversations in women's magazines about depression following childbirth. Throughout the 1970s and 1980s, depression became a more common topic, particularly in women's magazines and periodicals devoted to health. By the early 1990s, depression had become a common topic across different readership groups, including news magazines and general interest periodicals.[8] During the same time period that psychiatric researchers outlined a specific disease of depression through medication trials, symptom checklists, and research criteria, commentators in magazines warned Americans of the dangers of excessive sadness and the virtues of treatment. American readers became inundated with messages about depression as a "real disease," and based on the ongoing quantity of coverage of depression, they seemed to buy the idea.[9]

Through these discussions in popular magazines, physicians, social commentators, journalists, and readers shared a common language of depression by the end of the twentieth century. Physicians both wrote in popular magazines and applied contemporary social and cultural issues to their interpretations of epidemiological data.[10] Popular commentators invoked patient reports as well as physician expertise to define the problems of depression. And people who identified themselves as patients evaluated their options for acquiring help through their own efforts and through expert advice. Depression as a problem represented both individuals' struggles with the issues of everyday life and a serious psychiatric disorder that could require hospitalization—and at the worst might end in suicide. In its breadth of coverage and its significance for so many individuals, depression filled the places occupied by nervousness (common) and insanity (serious but less common) earlier in the century. Popular magazine readers were increasingly told that depression was something that could affect them—and that rising rates of depression were a serious national problem. For individual readers, depression became a way to articulate problems that would lead to some kind of consumption—pill, physician advice, or self-help technique. On a national level, depression became a grave threat to American optimism, particularly by the 1980s. The ultimate effect of the expanding conversation about depression was that unhappiness itself was transformed into a disease that could be treated. Evolving concepts of health and illness, along with commentators' concerns about national mood, meant that it was incumbent on all Americans to avoid sadness. With the modern concept of depression, the American creed of the pursuit of happiness took on a new and urgent meaning.[11]

Identifying the Problem

When reports of depression first appeared in American popular magazines in the late 1950s and 1960s, depression appeared to be an obscure, vaguely defined condition of relatively minor importance. In the 1960s, there were three times as many articles about anxiety as there were about depression, and many of the articles on depression were in women's magazines.[12] Even in television broadcast news of the time, "depression" was used more often to describe an economic condition than a mental state.[13] Yet by the 1980s coverage of depression in popular magazines had exploded, with frequent discussion of the illness in both general interest and news periodicals, and a large number of articles in both women's and health magazines. Over the decades, depression seemed to have greater and greater relevance to more and more readers, and appeared to become a major public health problem. Physicians, social commentators, and journalists participated in spreading the word about depression. In the process, they constructed a market for products that would be used to treat or prevent depression, particularly medications. By the 1980s, writers suggested that the most significant difficulty faced by most Americans was deciding when to get help for depression, not whether they were experiencing depressive symptoms.

At the time when magazine discussions of depression began to appear in women's periodicals in the 1960s, popular audiences had been exposed to increasing use of psychological—and even psychoanalytic—terminology to explain people's thoughts, feelings, and behavior.[14] Early articles on depression relied on the Freudian language of unconscious conflict and psychological stress.[15] But while psychological language initially helped to explain depression, the more lasting effect of American fluency in internal processes was to make emotional experiences a part of everyday reality. Further, internal experiences became defined as symptoms of disease that needed to be eradicated with treatment. Although the language of neurosis and reaction lingered in popular magazine accounts, by the 1970s depression was conceptualized as a disease—often with the implication that it was a process that derailed an otherwise functioning individual.[16]

Many Americans were first introduced to the idea of depression when it was revealed in 1972 that Missouri senator Thomas Eagleton, Democratic presidential candidate George McGovern's running mate, had been treated for "nervous" troubles. But though there was no formal psychiatric diagnosis of depression, Eagleton's difficulties were almost immediately labeled as depression by some members of the popular press, and writers and readers were alerted to the potential problems of the illness. To help engage readers, magazine writers employed the technique of addressing "you" the reader. For example, in 1972 Bertram Brown, the head of the National Institute of Mental Health (NIMH), was interviewed in an article titled "What You Should Know About Depression." In his remarks, Brown addressed the revelation about Senator Eagleton in terms of readers' possible experiences: "We would hope that through this and other examples more people now realize that you can have a severe depression, be hospitalized several times, and come back to full and effective functioning and enjoyment of life."[17] Writers suggested that depression could affect anyone.

Throughout the increasing popular discussions of depression in the rest of the 1970s and 1980s, writers—whether lay writers, physicians, or former patients—focused on the experience of feeling bad rather than on the ways in which a diagnosis of depression was made. Thus the transition to the formalized criteria of the third edition of *Diagnostic and Statistical Manual* (*DSM-III*) did not seem to significantly change magazine stories about depression. Instead, commentators stressed the distinction between negative feelings and "clinical" depression (though they did not say how to make the distinction), the importance of treatments, and the common nature of the disease. Though writers put significant energy into insisting that depression was real, counterarguments—minimizing the effects of depression—did not appear in mainstream American magazines.

Psychiatrists were frequently cited authorities on depression in popular magazines, and sometimes authored their own articles in their zeal to educate the public about the disease. For example, Gerald Klerman and Nathan Kline, physician researchers who were involved in medication trials that helped to develop the idea of depression, attempted to reach a broader audience by stepping outside of their usual peer publications and making contributions to popular magazines. Klerman and Kline, as well as other researchers in mental illness, appeared to be well-respected authorities in popular magazines by the 1970s. Some psychiatrists even wrote books to help patients deal with depression, a trend that has continued to accelerate.[18] Government authority also carried weight, as NIMH directors from Brown onward were frequently quoted and interviewed, and often answered questions about depression.[19] Psychiatrists were anxious to convey the information that depression was an increasingly important and easily treatable disease both inside and outside their own professional literatures.

Psychiatrists were not the only sources of information about depression, however. In the 1970s, several writers began to describe their personal encounters with depression in which they outlined their experiences as patients and as consumers of physician treatments and interventions.[20] Few patient writers gave all the credit for their recovery to a single intervention. *New York Times* correspondent Percy Knauth, for example, described his recovery from depression in the early 1970s as a combination of his efforts and those of his treating psychiatrists. Knauth summarized his experiences of treatment: "Not chemicals alone, not psychotherapy alone, but these treatments in combination are considered to be the most effective ways of curing depressive symptoms."[21]

Knauth and others who explained their depression did not deny the importance of treatment, but they framed the treatment in terms of their experiences
of consumers and the necessity of consulting multiple sources before finding
the right treatment.[22] Some writers emphasized that their knowledge of the
nature of depression, accumulated by reading books written by physicians on
the subject, helped them gain a sense of proportion and recovery from their
symptoms.[23] Others suggested that physicians faced serious deficits in their
ability to treat depression, and did not have a proper appreciation for treating
the whole person.[24] Writers stressed that depression was a real illness, analogous to other physical ailments. Not only was this a serious disease, but also it
could strike anyone—even readers of the magazines or their loved ones.

If depression was an actual disease, it should have some kind of physical
cause, and health-related periodicals emphasized the search for physical signs
and tests for depression. As first reported to the general public in *Psychology
Today* in 1974, investigators in depression had begun to look at neurotransmitters that were apparently affected by antidepressant medications.[25] Writers
characterized the theory of neurotransmitter deficits as a "chemical imbalance," a term used by journalists and psychiatrist-scientists alike. According
to the chemical imbalance theory, depression was caused by a deficiency in
a neurotransmitter (or two)—medication restored the levels of appropriate
neurotransmitters in the brain. The language of imbalance also connected to
the longer American tradition of nutritional deficiency that could be corrected
with vitamins.[26] By 1980, the explanation of depression as a chemical imbalance was in wide use in the American popular press. Writers emphasized
that patients needed to take medications, usually tricyclic antidepressants or
monoamine oxidase inhibitors (MAOIs), in order to correct the chemical imbalance and feel better.[27] Within this explanatory framework, depression sufferers
would fail to get better unless their chemicals had been properly adjusted.[28]
This theory of a chemical imbalance proved so compelling that it was used
to explain growing social problems, such as the rising divorce rate, which
was thought to be due to widespread untreated depression, conceptualized as
rampant, untreated chemical imbalance.[29]

The concept of imbalance within the body had wide resonance in American
popular culture in the second half of the twentieth century, and commentators
connected imbalance in the brain to other kinds of balance problems in bodily
functions. Depression could be imagined as a disruption of body rhythms—
especially in sleep and eating cycles. The chemical theory of depression could
expand beyond brain chemicals, as some speculated that depression was due
to other imbalances in nutrition or vitamins.[30] Commentators emphasized

that depression would result from disruptions in normal rhythms, but also suggested that modern conditions were not adequate to keep people from major emotional problems. For example, writers reported on a number of studies coming out of the NIMH on the theory of depression as a disorder caused by seasonal light changes, treated with light therapy.[31] The proper balance of light, food, and sleep was necessary to prevent or treat depression.

As general interest periodicals began to expand their coverage of depression by the 1980s, the concept of depression as a disease was often linked to physical signs or symptoms, as well as other diseases. Readers might encounter stories about tests for neurotransmitters and their metabolites in the blood and urine of patients, analogous to an X-ray to uncover depression.[32] Whether or not people could be definitively diagnosed, magazine readers were encouraged to think about depression if they thought that something was wrong with them. For example, health writers warned that viral infection or menopause was much less likely to cause emotional problems than depression, and that depression should be aggressively treated.[33] Further, the presence of depression could significantly affect physical ailments such as heart disease.[34] Depression had become an ailment inextricably tied to body function and chemistry, but also theoretically fixable by adjusting that body chemistry.[35]

By the late 1980s, millions of American readers of popular magazines were exposed to a plethora of stories about depression, its symptoms, its famous victims (especially Abraham Lincoln and Winston Churchill), and its treatment.[36] Further, readers encountered concrete, specific information about depression that stressed its status as a disease, possibly its biochemical mechanism, and definitely its treatment with specific medications. These discussions of depression not only emphasized the need to seek professional assistance (or some kind of self-help technique), but also they served to externalize sadness. The need to overcome sadness had important and far-reaching implications in the 1970s and 1980s.

Educating the Consumer about Depression

Popular magazine descriptions of depression focused on educating the consumer. Readers could obtain information on the nature of depression, advice about how to get out of a depressive episode by use of will power and/or a variety of activities, and encouragement to seek out further expert advice. Psychiatrists, who became frequent contributors to popular literature on this topic, also stressed surveillance for symptoms, as well as general exhortations to readers to consult professionals. All the information provided to readers about depression—whether self-help techniques or help-seeking activities—involved consumption. By conceptualizing depression as a problem for which readers/patients should seek expert advice *and* help themselves, writers significantly broadened the possible scope of people who might be affected by low mood and require some kind of intervention. Readers might be mildly depressed and require a new exercise routine (with new equipment) or a lunch out with a friend. Or they might need to buy books to help them with their mood management and maybe find a psychiatrist who could prescribe medication. As popular magazine stories covered a wide spectrum of depressive symptoms, from the blues to serious depression requiring hospitalization, readers received the information necessary to make educated consumer choices about the appropriate level of self-help or professional assistance.

For many who were thinking and writing about depression, the most logical connection between everyday experience and depression was the phenomenon of sadness around holidays and other ordinary experiences. Indeed, the ubiquity of these experiences helped introduce the concept of depression for general magazine audiences, particularly the idea of blues around holidays and vacations. As writers described the "normal" experiences of becoming sad during and after happy events, such as the winter holidays, childbirth, or occupational success, writers often provided mixed messages about sadness. On the one hand, they reassured readers that it was appropriate to occasionally have negative feelings. But at the same time, they also conveyed the message that these feelings needed to be eliminated through self-help or professional assistance.[37] During this time period, Americans were increasingly preoccupied with the self, including self-understanding and self-improvement, and were ready consumers for social and cultural discussions around self-help in the 1960s and 1970s, and even more so by the 1980s.[38]

While readers might readily identify with the experience of the blues at certain life transitions, the magazine portrayals of what needed to be done shifted over the decades. One lay writer argued in 1967 that normal people cycle in their moods and that it was important to work through sadness with specific activities.[39] Another writer reassured readers in 1970 that occasional bouts of sadness did not necessarily mean the onset of serious mental disease.[40] By the 1970s and 1980s, though, writers increasingly stressed the major problem of feeling sad. For example, "vacation blues" appeared to be times when people suffered what appeared to be inexplicable bouts of sadness—why should they be so sad when they were doing things that should make them happy?[41] Occasions for sad feelings provided writers an opportunity to explore the role of feelings in readers' lives.[42] But while negative feelings might be understandable, they were not to be tolerated. Writers shared tips for overcoming negative feelings, particularly by engaging in activities such as exercise.[43] American celebrities also participated in the popular magazine discussions of overcoming the blues by sharing their tricks for making themselves feel better.[44] Every December, a flood of writers shared tips for overcoming the holiday blues.[45] At the same time that readers participated in rituals of mass consumption, they were encouraged to strive to be happy while doing so and, if necessary, to consume in order to be happy to consume.[46]

Like the winter holidays, feelings of depression seemed to come around regularly, and popular commentators educated readers about symptoms and what to do to relieve them. Writers promoted self-help techniques and easily incorporated discussions of depression's severity along with cheerful, common-sense ways to deal with bad feelings. One writer in *McCall's* in 1983 described depression as something that "settles down over your world like a bad smell and gets into everything."[47] (Of course, American consumers by the 1980s knew how to prevent or eliminate smells!) Despite the bad smell, the author discouraged the use of medications or therapy and pointed out that people over the centuries had engaged in a variety of activities to help ease their depression, from baths to travel to distraction. While depression was a severe condition, the author likened it to a common cold: "Knowing it will come to an end, like a head cold, is a sort of therapy in itself."[48] As readers of *Reader's Digest* learned in 1983, they could use self-help and supportive measures to overcome the common experience of depression.[49]

While some authors used the metaphor of the bad cold and stressed ways in which readers could soothe themselves, other authors used much more frightening, dangerous metaphors to describe the risks of depression. What was a reader supposed to do? Was a person supposed to go to a doctor or deal with the problem himself or herself? If negative feelings were a normal response to stress, when would someone need a psychiatrist? The popular literature in the 1970s and 1980s never fully answered these questions, nor were not they clearly resolved in the medical literature either. Part of the problem in trying to help people determine when it was appropriate to seek out medical attention was that the advice about depression was spread out across all levels of severity. By providing such broad information, physicians and commentators emphasized the enormous prevalence of depressive symptoms and cast a broad net to capture the attention of anyone who might be suffering from depressive symptoms, however minor or severe. For example, Nathan Kline, one of the early researchers in antidepressant medication, wrote a popular book on depression that he explicitly stated was to help those who did not know they were depressed. For Kline and for others, the difficulty became how to empower people to change their lives while stressing that they needed treatment for a disease.[50]

Not all depression enthusiasts advocated medication, but it did comprise a major component of advice to readers in the popular literature.[51] As one author summarized in *McCall's* in 1972, "Whatever their view of the cause of depression, nearly all doctors, from general practitioners to psychiatrists, treat it the same way"—with medications.[52] For the most part, descriptions of medications for depression were fairly general: the two medication classes mostly commonly discussed were tricylic drugs and MAOIs. Few writers specifically mentioned brand-name medications, and most left the decision about when and how to medicate to physicians in consultation with their individual patients.[53] But writers' descriptions of medication use did not suggest that individuals who needed pharmaceutical intervention had failed. Instead, those who took medicine had an opportunity to join in a community of medication consumers.[54]

But medications were not the only forms of expert help available. The new psychotherapies that emerged by the late 1970s and 1980s appeared to provide a middle ground between self-help techniques and reliance on medications. As he explained in *Psychology Today* in 1977, psychiatrist Aaron Beck at the University of Pennsylvania developed a short-term, "commonsense" treatment of depression known as "cognitive therapy," which involved countering the negative thoughts in depressed people.[55] Beck was widely cited in the popular literature, and journalists and expert commentators stressed that Beck's therapy worked as well as—if not better than—medications.[56] His psychiatrist colleague David Burns published a popular book on cognitive therapy that was available to people working with therapists or on their own.[57] In addition to Beck's cognitive therapy, Yale psychiatrist Myrna Weissman and her colleagues developed Interpersonal Psychotherapy (IPT), another form of structured therapy that centered on working through difficulties in relationships.[58] These therapies were initially described primarily in health-related periodicals, but their ease of use and their promise for the future led to more widespread information about them in general periodicals. Commentators were excited about these therapies in the 1970s and 1980s, particularly because they were short term, inexpensive, and accessible to ordinary people (and might eliminate the need for medication for some patients).[59] In fact, one of the ways in which popular writers expressed their optimism about the ongoing progress in depression treatment was that it was no longer necessary to resort to the inexplicable, expensive, and prolonged process of psychoanalysis.[60]

Over the decades, popular magazine stories emphasized the ever-increasing number of treatments available for depression, from medications (initially MAOIs and tricyclic medications, and eventually Prozac, first mentioned in 1988) to short-term psychotherapy to other interventions such as light treatments for seasonal depression or exercise.[61] But the emergence of treatments for depression was not just a story of the expanding authority of experts. Instead, the growing number of methods to combat depression became part of a story of American progress and conquest over problems. One journalist in 1983 expressed this as a contrast between modern options and the hopeless suffering of depressed people of the past: "No longer are patients held hostage to the black moods and physical wasting away that crippled victims a generation ago."[62] By the late 1980s, writers cheerfully told the story of depression in terms of its many possible interventions—from medication to short-term focused psychotherapy to exercise to self-help techniques—that were available to all.[63] This optimism about depression treatments had clear implications for the nation's health.

America's Mental Health Issues

Depression did not gain currency in popular magazines just because it was a disease that could be treated. In the chaos and social upheavals of the 1960s and 1970s, depression made sense as a way to characterize the nation. In the 1970s in particular, depression seemed to characterize the national mood.[64] News and general interest writers picked up on the alarming estimates about the extent of depression, and many argued that the nation was going to suffer because of the wide extent of untreated illness. By the 1980s, though, the story of depression had a more optimistic turn. Instead of wailing about the negative consequences of increasing depression, commentators began to describe the story of depression as an optimistic lesson about scientific achievement. Yes, depression was prevalent and costly. But at the same time, modern science in psychiatry was tackling the threat. All that was needed was further national investment in the research efforts of American psychiatrists.

Even as writers explained treatment for individuals, many of the general interest periodicals from the 1970s on kept up a running commentary about the American mood and the implications of depression on the national population and character. According to *Newsweek* in 1973, depression was taking on the characteristics of an epidemic and was threatening to sweep the nation.[65] In the early 1970s, stories in *Harper's Bazaar* and the *New York Times Magazine* indicated that between eight and ten million Americans needed treatment for depression, although they currently were not receiving it. Indeed, the *New York Times Magazine* article identified depression as the "common cold" of mental ailments, a metaphor used to emphasize its ubiquity in America.[66] In 1975, *Good Housekeeping* reported that nineteen million Americans were suffering from depression, while a *Saturday Evening Post* account the same year claimed that approximately twenty million Americans had current symptoms of depression, and that half of the population would eventually suffer from depression at one time in their lives.[67] A writer for *Good Housekeeping* claimed that eight million Americans would seek treatment for depression over the next year, while thirty-two million would suffer without treatment.[68] The highest estimate of depression in the general population during these decades was a report in *Intellect* in 1977 that sixty million Americans were depressed.[69] In 1978, Aaron Beck reported in *Psychology Today* that 78 percent of college students were going to become depressed during the next academic year.[70]

The alarming estimates of the growing numbers of depressed people in the population during the 1970s seemed to reflect a national sense that something had gone terribly wrong with American society, particularly for the nation's youth. As Dr. Joyce Brothers explained in *Good Housekeeping* in 1971, "These are stressful times. Vietnam, student unrest, racial tensions, urban decay, the threat of pollution and overpopulation . . . all create an air of impending crisis."[71] *Newsweek* writers explained that younger people were particularly susceptible to the social problems of the day: "There is some evidence that depression is spreading most rapidly among the nation's young people. Some psychiatrists discern a pervasive apathy among American youth, produced they believe, by frustration over the war and the environment and confusion over social values."[72] As another writer pointed out, "The 1960s was a decade of rebellion among young people. Researchers categorize the 1970s as the era of depression."[73] In these discussions, causes and consequences merged as writers concluded that social upheaval should be addressed by diagnosing and treating depression in the nation's youth.

Some explicitly suggested that the 1970s youth crisis was due to some kind of social or environmental agent that predisposed younger people to serious depression.[74] A physician explained in *Harper's Bazaar* that a loss of enjoyment, feelings of fatigue, and a tendency to complain characterized "the social disease of the '70s—low-grade, chronic depression."[75] In 1979, Gerald Klerman wrote that the 1970s had become the "Age of Melancholy," especially for the nation's youth.[76] Klerman and others speculated that young people of the Baby Boom generation, who had come of age at a time when opportunities for young people were scarcer than they had come to expect, were suffering from depression related to impossible expectations. Further, growing economic troubles in the nation and increased social isolation were likely to precipitate an increase in the rate of depression.[77]

The culture of the 1980s seemed to provide a foil to the malaise and depression of the 1970s. The optimism and hope expressed by President Ronald Reagan signaled to many a new positive outlook in the nation. While some critics suggested that Reagan-era optimism was just a cover for Americans' inability to tolerate the empty consumer drive that dominated their lives, most commentators accepted the optimism at face value and embraced the idea that happiness was a national goal.[78] Cultural optimism provided not only a rationale for treatment for depression but also helped to characterize popular discussions of the ailment. Depression appeared to be common (and perhaps even increasing), but it could be easily treated, particularly through wise consumption—especially of medical resources.

But though depression was a national problem, there were some portions of the population that seemed to be at greater risk. Popular magazine discussions about the role of depression in the United States often focused on the dangers to children and adolescents of the disease, echoing television news reports that also stressed the dangers to teenagers from suicide.[79] As a writer for *Teen* explained in 1980, "Suicide attempts are up tenfold since the end of World War II, particularly among young people. Prescription drugs for depression fill medicine cabinets across the country. Self-help books on feeling better consistently make the bestseller list. Literally millions of Americans are caught in the grip of serious depression, and teenagers are part of that group."[80] The fact that so many people were taking medications and engaging in self-help for depression pointed to the growing magnitude of the problem. The troubles of youth in the early 1980s, as one commentator explained, were a legacy of the turmoil of the 1970s: "The era of Vietnam, Watergate, several assassinations, the 'me' generation, liberalized sexual mores, widespread abuse of drugs and alcohol, and the glorification of violence in movies and on TV was bound to take its toll."[81] By the late 1980s, journalists and psychiatrists were speculating about an "agent blue," some cultural or environmental factor that seemed to have the effect of increasing depression in youth.[82]

Yet at the same time that the nation's youth appeared to be in serious danger, many popular accounts—particularly in magazines directed at teenagers—emphasized that depression was part of normal growth. As one writer in *Seventeen* explained in 1978, "Depression, for a large percentage of young people, is part of the teen years, as common as sweating over finals, having a crush on a rock star, or needing to borrow the family car."[83] Although articles such as this one cited physician authorities, including Nathan Kline, the message for teenage readers was optimistic. And while these articles did mention that teenagers needed to get help for serious depression, they offered advice to teens for overcoming their negative feelings.[84]

While teenagers appeared particularly vulnerable to depression, older adults also came under scrutiny for what some perceived as their vulnerability to depression. By the late 1970s and early 1980s, commentators began to describe a growing problem of depression—as well as a host of other medical and emotional issues—among older people.[85] Not coincidentally, during this time period products and services for retired individuals also began to proliferate, including magazines directed at seniors. These magazines emphasized that depression was common in older people, as one *Retirement Living* article in 1977 estimated that about one in four over the age of sixty-five suffered from depression.[86] But while depression in adolescence seemed to be part of growing up, the issue of normal depression in old age was more problematic. Some writers exhorted aging individuals to be on the constant lookout for depression, but others expressed confidence that older people could deal with it. A research group explained in 1985 that severe depression was actually less common in older people and that older folks were more resilient: "We hope that these findings will counteract the negative stereotypes, held by many professionals and elders alike, concerning an older person's capacity to change and grow."[87] The authors emphasized that older people were not necessarily more prone to depression and also suggested that psychotherapy was better than medications for this population. This research group emphasized that older people got better, not that older people did not get depressed in the first place.

Not all the magazine descriptions of elderly depression were defensive, though. Some pointed out that there were potential positives of depression. An author in *Retirement Living* in 1975 argued that depression was an opportunity for growth, particularly for older people.[88] Others emphasized that famous individuals such as Winston Churchill had suffered from depression.[89] Further, a number of writers reported on studies done by researchers Kay Jamison and Nancy Andreasen that suggested that mental illness was correlated with heightened creativity. Perhaps, authors speculated, the rising rates of depression might actually bring with them outpourings of creative talent.[90] Still, the elderly remained a group that needed special attention during the aging process, particularly in terms of surveillance for depression.

By the 1980s, estimates of the numbers of depressed people had become somewhat less alarming compared to the 1970s estimates, but journalists

followed the lead of the scientists they were quoting and continued to emphasize the magnitude of the problem in terms of percentages of the population
and the burden of the illness. In the medical literature, the numbers could
be enormous. One psychiatrist in 1981 claimed that "as much as half of the
population can be expected to have a serious depressive episode at some
point in their lives."[91] In comparison, the estimates in the popular literature
varied widely, from a 1984 *FDA Consumer* speculation that approximately 3
to 4 percent of the American population were depressed at any one time, to a
claim in 1985 that there were nine million "victims" of depression annually.[92]
Writers in the United States emphasized that this was not the only country
affected by the overwhelming increase in depression. As a *World Press Review*
article in 1984 explained, 100 million people developed "recognizable depression" worldwide every year.[93]

Popular writers echoed and amplified concerns about depression that
had been articulated by psychiatrists such as Alan Stoudemire about the
costs of depression.[94] But popular representations of depression went beyond
cost to emphasize the ways in which depression affected U.S. culture. In the
magazine literature in the United States between the 1960s and 1990s, depression appeared prevalent, responsible for a tremendous social and economic
burden, and problematic in terms of American life. But at the same time that
commentators warned of the burden of depression, they also pointed out
that depression was responsive to treatment. Many provided easy answers
to the major national problem of depression, to encourage more individuals
to consume products that would help them. As commentators increasingly
pointed out in the 1980s, bad feelings were costly to the nation.

Depression's Expanding Boundaries

As advocates educated the public about the extent and risks of untreated
depression, the definitions of depression became more broad and more inclu-
sive. Further, a sense of urgency began to apply to all cases, from relatively
mild to severe—with the often-stated assumption that hidden depression of any
kind could and would result in suicide. Educators expressed genuine worry
about an outcome as terrible as suicide, but they also blurred the distinctions
between sadness and depression, distinctions that became almost meaningless
by the early 1990s. In the 1970s, social commentators were alarmed about the
extent of depression and suffering, and attributed much of it to the upheavals
in the previous decades. But at the same time, popular culture during that
decade seemed to accommodate a certain amount of sadness as part of life.[95]
By the 1980s, however, the social, cultural, and political culture had shifted to

make expressions of sadness appear to be pathological in and of themselves. In this climate, feeling sad was something to overcome.

As information about depression first began to circulate in the popular literature, commentators often made a rhetorical distinction between mild and serious depression. For example, the NIMH's Bertram Brown explained in 1974 that "clinically, we mean something more serious when we speak of depression. In the intermediate stage, victims feel a lack of energy and interest in life that hangs on for a few days or a few weeks and affects their life functions."[96] As information about depression became more widespread, though, it appeared increasingly difficult to distinguish between sadness and "clinical" depression.[97] Further, the potential for suicide was frightening enough to suggest that more people should be treated, regardless of the apparent severity of their symptoms. Although most of the sociological literature on suicide prior to this time did not identify depression (or other psychiatric diagnosis) as a particular factor in suicide, the common wisdom in popular magazines by the 1970s was that untreated depression could and would result in suicide.[98] One physician pointed out in 1964 that more than 20,000 people died every year from suicide and that more than a third of them were depressed.[99] Another physician stated in *Vogue* in 1972 that depression was in fact the reason that people killed themselves.[100] A *New York Times Magazine* article in 1979 about depression in children was dramatically titled "Catching Them Before They Suicide."[101] These authors and others asserted that it was imperative for the nation's health to increase the treatment of depression and reduce the risk for suicide.[102]

But while suicide prevention provided one motive to treat depression, others suggested that it was important to treat depression in order to eliminate suffering. As Roy Menninger, the president of the psychoanalytic Menninger Foundation, explained in 1978, "there has been too much of a tendency in both medicine and psychiatry to be concerned only with the seriously ill, and not to consider these problems of living as part of their bailiwick. As a result, a lot of people have gone elsewhere in search of quick and easy solutions."[103] Although most of the psychiatrists and therapists quoted or interviewed by the 1980s did not share Menninger's psychoanalytic views, they did validate the idea that all varieties of suffering deserved to be treated.[104]

As writers increasingly described sadness as a problem that needed and deserved treatment, the category of depression as a disease began to expand, and the circumstances under which individuals might be expected to become depressed appeared more common. For example, *Psychology Today* writers reported that researchers had identified major life stresses (such as the death of a spouse) that were more likely to lead to depression. But rather than limit their attention to those individuals who experienced major stresses, researchers noted that patients' negative perception of their lives was more important than the actual objective measure of adverse events in their lives.[105] Further, other *Psychology Today* writers commented on research that illustrated that it was actually depressing to be around depressed people.[106] Writers in women's magazines picked up on this theme and described friends with depression and how, despite their wish to help, it could be dangerous to someone's mental health to get too close to a depressed person.[107] Depression was not just an epidemic for its immediate victims; it could conceivably spread as depressed people drew others down into their depression.

Depression as a disease expanded in the 1980s as writers, echoing and magnifying research literature, began to describe the broad spectrum of depressive conditions, especially mood problems that were significant because of their longevity rather than their severity. A number of writers began to describe phenomena of low-grade chronic depression, or dysthymia, and framed this in terms of increasing help available to larger portions of the population. As one journalist explained in *New York* in 1986, "Scientific attention once focused almost exclusively on one end of the spectrum—depression that is almost totally incapacitating. But now scientists are finally paying attention to a long-ignored, less flamboyant form of the illness—chronic mild depression."[108] First-person and journalist accounts of chronic mild depression emphasized that it was devastating to the victim and previously ignored by the scientific community. But while its advocates pointed to its prevalence in American society, the definitions of chronic mild depression were so vague that they could include anyone who felt badly for a long time for any reason.[109]

In response to the reported epidemic of depression among younger people, a number of parenting magazines began to include advice to parents about how to deal with their depressed youngsters.[110] As some writers pointed out, depressive symptoms in children began to achieve new significance to psychiatrists by the 1980s, but parents perceived professional disagreement about whether children suffered from a "clinical" depression or how to diagnose it.[111] Parents were encouraged to help with this process, educate their children about dealing with their emotions, and seek out expert advice about whether their children needed psychiatric attention.[112] But in addition, parents learned that their own untreated (or inadequately treated) depression could worsen their children's symptoms.[113] Depression was a problem not just in individuals but also in their relationships and in the broader society as a whole.

Perhaps depression was a problem of society itself? Nathan Kline argued in 1975 that the large number of untreated sufferers of depression was not surprising—they probably did not believe they had the right to be happy. As he explained, American culture was still somewhat Puritan, and stoic Americans still assumed that suffering was good, an attitude that led depressed individuals to avoid treatments such as medication.[114] But commentators argued by the 1980s that it was not good to see suffering as valuable. Several psychological studies in the 1980s pointed out that students with mild depression predicted the world and likely outcomes for themselves more realistically than their nondepressed colleagues. But rather than see this realistic outlook as positive or desirable, psychologists concluded that the comparably more rosy view of the world of nondepressed people needed to be studied further in order to provide a model for preventing depression.[115] By this time, no longer did Americans believe that denial and hardship were necessary conditions. Instead, it appeared to be possible—and necessary—to eliminate unhappiness altogether.[116]

The move toward pathologizing unhappiness did not go without comment, however, as not everyone agreed that eradicating unhappiness was a laudable goal. In 1984, New York psychologist Lesley Hazleton argued that the national move toward depression had reduced the range of acceptable feelings in Americans. As a *Time* review explained, "Hazleton's view of depression is simple enough: she says that it is overpsychologized and overmedicated. Her book argues that ordinary sadness and an occasional bout of the blues are now routinely given the psychiatric label 'depression,' and anyone admitting to bad feelings is in danger of being hustled off for a so-called cure through therapy or drugs."[117] For Hazleton, the problem was not just that there was too much emphasis on depression, but also that the culture had become intolerant of negative feelings. A few others also argued that depression was an important response to life situations that needed to be learned from rather than just overcome.[118]

Martin Seligman, a psychologist who was best known for his theory that depression represented a state of learned helplessness, explained in 1988 that American society's emphasis on the individual made it more likely that the individual was going to internalize distress and become depressed. Bad things happen to people, but "the new emphasis on the self raises the chances that we will blame these misfortunes, losses and disappointments on ourselves and thus depress ourselves."[119] While Seligman saw depression as a problem, he suggested that people seek out the common good in their communities and avoid preoccupation with their own internal issues.

In their efforts, though, advocates for the importance of sadness had to contend with psychiatrists such as Robert Hirschfeld, the director of NIMH, who in 1987 insisted that depression was a medical illness (with both biochemical and psychological factors).[120] Hazelton's and Seligman's voices were largely drowned out by the proliferation of products and services and well-meaning educational efforts designed to help treat and prevent depression. For most commentators by the 1990s, depression was a major public health problem—and it had readily available consumer solutions including medications and other kinds of methods to deal with unhappiness, such as "learning vacations" to help people overcome loss or disappointment.[121] In an effort to avoid depression, Americans were encouraged to avoid all bad feelings and to rely on external assistance to experience normal changes in life.

Commentators and educators in the area of depression made it clear that depression was a major problem in American society and that individuals needed to learn about the symptoms and the treatments. Instead of viewing unhappiness as a natural result of life experiences, popular magazine coverage stressed that unhappiness was likely caused by an external process. The presentation of unhappiness as a disease in need of a treatment was reinforced by magazine portrayals of individuals who described their depression treatments in terms of consumption.[122] In some ways, this information helped to demystify the illness as the revelations about celebrities gave new visibility to depression as an illness in the 1980s.[123] But celebrity accounts of depression sometimes appeared similar to endorsements of consumer products over the decades in the twentieth century: depression could be seen as a condition for which readily available commodities could be purchased.[124]

In 1990, science journalist Erica Goode explained in *U.S. News and World Report* that depression was still a subject of embarrassment for victims, but was gradually becoming more accepted as an important problem: "Though it is more common than diabetes, serious depression—the kind that can lead to suicide or land one in a mental hospital—remains an issue that can unhorse presidential candidates or bind a family in an embarrassed silence. There are signs, however, that this view is shifting, that science is at last making headway against fear."[125] Goode's article nicely summed up the major advances of the previous decades, and she highlighted the importance of drug treatments, psychotherapy, and the increased incidence in younger people. She cited many of the most important figures in studies of depression of the time, and also described some of the increasingly sophisticated scientific theories around the neurochemical abnormalities that were implicated in depression.

Goode's article suggested that the relatively recent widespread awareness of depression's seriousness was due to physician discoveries and new treatments. Goode and other writers emphasized that public understanding and further education would continue to make headway against the vast numbers of undiagnosed and untreated depressed patients. But the story of evolving discussions about depression has not just been about the transfer of medical information to the public or the generation of new knowledge. Instead, the widespread awareness of depression as an illness in the last decades of the twentieth century has been a part of a process of commodifying depression and offering consumers choices in treatments.[126] While there are certainly groups who make money from promoting depression as an illness, this promotion has not necessarily been driven by self-interest. Instead, advocates sincerely believe that Americans need to know more about depression in order to prevent national catastrophe.

In the popular literature in the second half of the twentieth century, depression became an important and compelling way to express distress on an individual and social level. While many articles by the 1980s included specific criteria for psychiatrist-diagnosed depression, most authors (including physicians) used the concept of depression more broadly to encompass a variety of problems. Psychiatrists defined a disease entity of depression to be consistent across treatment and research sites. Depression in the public sphere, however, had a broader role as the language of depression allowed writers to explain problems and articulate solutions (medication, psychotherapy, self-help, or some combination of the three). Depression was not just a way of pathologizing conditions; it was also a way of framing problems in a manner that allowed for an easy and readily available solution. If the malaise in American society was due to widespread depression, it would be easy to treat—presumably, all we need is more diagnosis and more treatment of the illness. And we need to consume more products in order to help treat the depression. Indeed, the concept of depression itself has become an object of consumption as depression educational guides have become a staple in bookstores, including perhaps the inevitable *Depression for Dummies*.[127]

But as depression expanded as a diagnosis and a cultural construct over the past few decades, it has not been described as a problem that equally affects men and women. Instead, over the past few decades most of the articles in both medical and magazine literature have stated or assumed that depression is a particular problem for women. In discussions about depression, women have been targeted as objects of medical inquiry and also solicited as sophisticated consumers of products and medical services. As a result, depression itself has been shaped around the perceived issues and needs of women.

Chapter 4

Gender, Depression, Diagnosis, and Power

One of the most commonly reported "facts" about depression is that it is at least twice as common in women as it is in men. Modern researchers have speculated on the possible causes for this difference. While some have raised questions about women's social and economic vulnerability that might lead them to become more depressed, others have looked for explanations within women's brains, particularly for correlations to the biological feature in which women are the most different from men: their reproductive hormones. Depression as we know it now is definitely diagnosed more in women than in men. But is that because of women or because of the way depression is defined?

Psychiatrists and other physicians have a long history of using biology to explain women's social and emotional problems. In 1899, for example, Minnesota's Saint Peter State Hospital superintendent H. A. Tomlinson warned that women in America were in grave danger from insanity because they were "warring against their natural position" of bearing children and attempting to avoid responsibility through their grasping for "material advancement or social opportunity."[1] Tomlinson's bombasts echoed other late-nineteenth-century physicians who insisted that women's modern strivings were violations of their biological destiny. Like many physicians of his time (as well as before and after), Tomlinson structured his theories about the origins of women's illness (in this case, insanity) within assumptions about women's appropriate gender roles as embedded within their biological systems.

As is easy to see from the distance of time, pronouncements such as Tomlinson's clearly reflected (and likely reinforced) prevailing discomfort with women's new social roles at the turn of the century.[2] Tomlinson, like other physicians before and since, conflated women's biological sex with their social and cultural roles, expectations based on gender.[3] But not only did psychiatrists like Tomlinson project historically contingent gender roles onto women's biological attributes, they did so within psychiatric institutions. For patients and psychiatrists in the early twentieth century, gender dynamics involved not just physician descriptions of gender role violations but also the power dynamic of hospitalization.[4]

Over the course of the twentieth century, though, psychiatrists gradually moved away from enacting gender assumptions through lengthy psychiatric hospital stays, while their pronouncements about gender roles became less crude or obviously sexist. Medical explanations that relied on reference to patient sex did not disappear, however. The disease of depression as it emerged in medical discussions in the second half of the twentieth century was based on deeply embedded gender assumptions, disguised within the biological language of sex. But unlike earlier disease descriptions based on gender about which women sometimes made objections, depression as a disease primarily of women involved agreement between physicians and patients within a comfortable scientific framework. While critics have been vocal in their protest about the gender assumptions in other psychiatric diseases with a lopsided sex ratio, the idea that depression is a disease more common in women has been accepted by those concerned about women and mental health, even for those who otherwise question psychiatric authority.[5]

How did psychiatrists come to the conclusion that depression was a disease that occurred mostly in women? How is the diagnosis itself gendered? And finally, why do women accept the idea that depression is a women's disease? It is clear that gender assumptions have been and continue to be present in psychiatric theory and practice, particularly in the emergence of depression. While the language, tone, and intent have changed, physicians are still telling women that they are controlled by their biological destiny. But now physicians have found a way to say it that seems to make sense to large numbers of American women who have bought the idea that brain chemistry gone awry is the reason for their troubles.

Gender and Mental Disease

In the first half of the twentieth century, psychiatrists and neurologists assumed that men and women had specific roles in society, and professionals frequently explained mental disease or distress in terms of problems with these roles. Although physicians employed gender language, they assumed that all differences between men and women were based in biology. The binary distinction between male and female helped to structure their ideas about patients as well as their medical practice. Gender roles became particularly codified and extended with the rise of psychoanalysis and its popularization in the mental hygiene movement. Within its theoretical framework, men or women who strayed outside of their roles could be vulnerable to mental disease.

Psychiatrists often used descriptions of sex differences to illustrate their understandings of mental disease, and their constant awareness of a patient's sex throughout all descriptions of patient problems and treatments reveals the critical role that sex (and gender) played in their thinking. Psychiatrists and neurologists worked in hospitals and clinics in which the binary distinction between men and women was a fact of life. At a time when other categories of difference—including race, class, and ethnicity—were frequently the subject of intense public discussion, sex appeared comfortably self-evident. Though physicians remained convinced that sex differences were biological, what they ascribed to sex changed throughout the century. In addition, the diseases that captured psychiatrists' attention shifted over time with changing social, cultural, and professional contexts. Early in the century, women were more likely to be treated for hysteria, while men were more often treated for neurasthenia. A few decades later, psychiatrists made efforts to describe and treat involutional melancholia, a constellation of emotional and physical problems that occurred around the climacteric that seemed to be most prominent in women.

American psychiatrists and neurologists in the first half of the twentieth century made a point of including sex in their descriptions of patient populations and linked sex to diagnosis. In 1906, for example, prominent New York neurologist Smith Ely Jelliffe characterized the dispensary population he was treating and noted that he saw a large population of neurasthenic patients in a year's time—393 cases, of which 248 were men and 145 were women. He also noted that he saw 106 cases of hysteria, of which 8 were men and 98 were women. Jelliffe commentated on the sex ratio difference between neurasthenia and hysteria, and admitted that the same patient's symptoms were likely to be classified under neurasthenia for men and hysteria for women.[6] Yet rather than interpret this as a problem with diagnosis, Jelliffe accepted that it was part of the difference between men and women.[7]

In the early twentieth century, men in particular appeared to be vulnerable to nervous disorders because of rapid changes within the American work environment.[8] Physicians cautioned that men endangered themselves if they became too deeply enmeshed in work in response to the transition from small, face-to-face business communities to larger bureaucratic organizations.

As New York hospital physician Warren Babcock described in 1900, the consequence of overwork was nervousness: "In the average business man, who voluntarily subjects himself to an intolerable grind of office work, without adequate exercise, the development of neurasthenic symptoms, so often the antecedent of melancholia, should be the first indication for preventive treatment."[9] Of course, men could also develop neurasthenia if they did not work enough.[10] In the early twentieth century, the average businessman's health and efficiency were of vital importance to politicians, health activists, and Progressive-era reformers. Efficiency standards of the time dictated that there was an optimal quantity and quality of work. Maintaining a balance between work and leisure, therefore, was not just a problem for the individual but was also a problem for the American economy as a whole.[11]

Although neurasthenia seemed to affect men through work stress, women appeared to be vulnerable to hysteria.[12] Hysteria as a diagnosis had reached its heyday in the late nineteenth century, but American physicians at the beginning of the twentieth century still incorporated aspects of older ideas of female hysteria within new diagnostic groupings.[13] By the early twentieth century, psychiatrists criticized older methods of treatment, particularly Philadelphia neurologist S. Weir Mitchell's nineteenth-century rest cure, but they retained the desire to enforce a gendered power dynamic with their patients. Their attempts to assert power, however, were not always successful. As early psychoanalytic enthusiast Ernest Jones pointed out in 1913, hysterical patients were likely to be hypersensitive to the words of their physicians: "Any such may serve to produce a radical change in the patient's attitude toward him, to lead to respect being replaced by antipathy, irritation, dread, hate, or—most troublesome of all—affection. It is this fickle behavior of hysterical patients that often leads physicians to regard the treatment of them as an ungrateful task, to be avoided whenever possible."[14] Psychiatrists' frustrations with their hysterical patients' refusal to be passive, especially their "fickle behavior," structured descriptions of the disease as well as the treatment.

But even as neurasthenia and hysteria were eclipsed by other diagnoses, psychiatrists and neurologists continued to employ fundamental distinctions between men and women in their descriptions of patient populations. In his 1913 textbook, Philadelphia neurologist Francis Dercum asserted that manic-depressive insanity occurred twice as frequently in women than in men.[15] New York statistician Horatio Pollack reported in 1925 that men in cities were more frequently admitted to New York hospitals, although women in cities formed a larger proportion of the patients diagnosed with manic-depression and involutional melancholia. Pollack speculated that men were particularly vulnerable to the stresses and strains of urban life.[16] He noted, however, that men and women appeared to be equally likely to suffer a recurrence of manic-depressive psychosis.[17] An office-based psychiatrist in Washington, D.C., pointed out in 1934 that milder depression seen in office settings was as common in men as in women, although women predominated in the more severe cases in the hospital.[18] While some demographic details were recorded more regularly than others, the sex distribution of patients was a reliable feature of these early efforts at mental health statistics. Physicians and statisticians assumed that the sex ratios for mental illness were essential to the scientific gathering of information in the field.[19] Indeed, psychiatrists were much more consistent about the importance of differences between the sexes than they were about which diagnoses were more prevalent in which sex.[20]

Even though there was no clear pattern of sex predominance in any one category of mental illness, psychiatrists were convinced that sex role violations could and would lead to insanity for both men and women.[21] In the first few decades of the century, psychiatrists frequently focused on the importance of these roles, especially within an increasingly psychoanalytic framework.[22] Psychoanalytic views of men and women were not hegemonic during this time period or after.[23] But psychiatrists and neurologists, particularly within the mental hygiene movement, put existing gender roles into a therapeutic language. Violation of these norms was by definition pathological, and mental disease could be expected to be both evidence and cause of gender role problems.

But gender roles did not remain static over time for either American society or individual women. The early-twentieth-century diagnosis of involutional melancholia, which was tied throughout its history to changing roles for women, illustrates the shifts in role expectations. Although involutional melancholia had originally been described by Emil Kraepelin in the context of late-nineteenth-century German hospital populations, it was popular among American psychiatrists (and neurologists) because it seemed to capture both biology and American understandings of pathology surrounding gender role violations.[24] Involutional melancholia, a pattern of disordered mood, behavior, and thinking that seemed to occur in the years around the climacteric (tied explicitly to menopause in women in their forties and fifties, but less anchored for men in their fifties and sixties), was originally debated by American psychiatrists at the beginning of the century but achieved a particular significance by the time of the rise of the somatic therapies in the 1940s.

For centuries, psychiatrists had presumed a connection between women's reproductive apparatus and their mental health.[25] Early-twentieth-century physicians linked melancholic symptoms with menstruation and/or child-birth.[26] One Ohio physician explained in 1901 that melancholia had "been attributed to the influence of the various diseases incident to menstruation, lactation and the numerous disorders of pregnancy."[27] Another assistant physician at an asylum studied a population of patients with manic-depressive psychosis to try to understand the intervals between attacks of illness in seventy-four women and thirty-one men. He found that prognosis appeared to be worse when the attacks appeared in close relationship to menstrual disorders.[28] Most psychiatrists accepted as a matter of course that mental illness in women was connected to their unique biology. As they tracked the numbers of men and women, these professionals assumed that differences in expression of mental illness and outcome of treatment between men and women were directly due to their biological differences.[29]

Some within psychiatry were aware that early-twentieth-century medical views of women perhaps overdetermined the role of their reproductive cycles, and for this they blamed the other specialty that took care of women, gynecology.[30] In 1903, Washington, D.C., psychiatrist William A. White commented that gynecologists were too enthusiastic about abdominal operations to treat mental disease in women: "Our misguided friend the gynecologist . . . has insisted that all forms whatsoever of mental disease affecting the female were traceable to an affection of the uterus or its appendages, and has devised all manner of operations to relieve such conditions. . . . But the sort of stuff that mind is made of is not to be found in the abdominal cavity."[31] Although White blamed gynecologists for the overemphasis on women's biology, many psychiatrists and neurologists were unwilling to let go of what seemed to them self-evident ties between women's cycles and their mental illness.

But though menstrual function appeared an obvious component of involutional melancholia, psychiatrists easily moved back and forth between reference to hormones and reference to problems with psychological function. Indeed, for these professionals there was no distinction between biology and other determinants of women's lives. According to many physicians, older women were vulnerable to problems in later life through emotional, family, social, and economic stresses. In 1912, Rochester State Hospital psychiatrist E. P. Ballentine summarized the causes of involutional melancholia in terms of the difficulties with women's roles: "The exciting etiological factors were ill health, including derangements incident to the climacteric, shock from death of near relatives—often augmented by strain of nursing during the final illness—business reverses, financial worries, difficulties connected with making a living, privation and overwork."[32] Early descriptions of involutional melancholia stressed the sheer magnitude of the problems facing elderly patients, a population that was significantly increasing in psychiatric hospitals in the early twentieth century.[33] With this many strains, psychiatrists were not at all surprised that many older women seemed to fall victim to involutional melancholia.

Not only did older women have to deal with external stresses, but also internal conflicts appeared to be overwhelming at this time of life. One woman physician explained in 1925 that involutional melancholia was particularly common in people who could not adjust to their advancing age: "It is the men and women who have failed to develop broad interests and to establish contacts outside the home or business circle who appear to be especially prone to agitated depressions. Often they have lived exemplary lives, been efficient and achieved a measure of success, yet a certain inelasticity of temperament militates against their acceptance of the declining phase of life."[34] Although appropriate gender roles determined how individuals should live their lives, psychiatrists cautioned that too rigid an adherence to these roles (as well as abandonment of them altogether) could be harmful. According to psychiatrists, acceptance of decline in later years was critical to prevent patients from fleeing reality into psychosis.[35]

While many psychiatrists suggested that internal conflicts and external events predisposed individuals to involutional melancholia, psychoanalytically oriented practitioners developed even more sophisticated theoretical constructs for the issues faced by elderly women. As Baltimore psychiatrist Eleanora Saunders pointed out, menopausal patients "drift easily into ruminations of loss, of self-censure, of regret, and of guilt because of neglected opportunity in past life, because of doubts of the present, and of feelings of personal inadequacy for the future. They may, with the waning of the biological drive at the involutional period, react to frustration or loss with deeper and more enduring depression than was characteristic for them in the depressive reactions of the earlier years."[36] The language of adjustment, which helped psychoanalysts articulate their concerns during this time period, was useful in helping to explain the problems of older women (and sometimes men) as they aged.[37] Not only psychoanalysts but also psychiatrists of all theoretical perspectives utilized the concepts of adjustment and personality to make sweeping generalizations about aging people, particularly women, and their problems with mental illness in old age.[38]

In order to develop their ideas about the relationship between mental disease and gender identity, psychiatrists looked to the field of psychology, where such inquiries had led to specific tests by the 1930s.[39] During the

1930s and 1940s, Stanford psychologists Louis Terman and Catherine Miles quantified male and female characteristics through the "M.F. test" (masculinity/femininity), which could help assess individuals and their deviations from the norm.[40] Psychiatrists Beulah Bosselman and Bernard Skorodin at the University of Illinois used the M.F. test on psychiatric patients with the rationale that, since psychiatric patients were socially maladjusted, they would likely be maladjusted in their sex roles as well. The M.F. test illustrated correlations that expressed 1930s ideas about male and female gender roles, sexual expression, and aggression: "Intelligence was found to correlate positively with masculinity in women; there was no such relationship shown in men. Overt male passive homosexuals had highly feminine scores; a small series of overt female active homosexuals had masculine scores." The researchers concluded that male schizophrenic patients were found to deviate to the feminine, while female schizophrenic and manic-depressive patients deviated (although less so) to the masculine.[41] Sex role problems were not just incidental to the disease, but in fact appeared to help define the pathology.

In the 1930s and 1940s, psychiatrists' conviction about the importance of sex roles led them to try to prevent involutional melancholia in older women through intervention with women in their younger years. In particular, professionals identified women's narrow areas of interest as a potential problem in later life.[42] According to psychiatrists interested in prevention, women invested too much energy in their children and then had no other activities to keep them occupied when their children left home. But of course the exhortation to women to develop other interests conflicted with psychiatrists' constant message that children needed their mothers' undivided attention in order to prevent major mental problems later in life.[43]

At the same time that psychiatrists constructed a double bind for women based on their interactions with their children, a number of psychiatrists fell back on ties between menopause and mental symptoms that made involutional melancholia appear to be a clear-cut case of a biologically based illness. Not all American psychiatrists embraced involutional melancholia and its connection to women's hormones, nor did they explicitly exclude men. But much of the literature on the illness centered on women and biological interventions.[44] For example, New York psychiatrists August Hoch and John MacCurdy carefully analyzed sixty-seven cases of involutional melancholia to understand the important symptoms—twenty-two of the cases were men, forty-five of the cases were women.[45] New Orleans psychiatrist Frank Fenwick Young explained that involutional melancholia was five times more common in women than in men, likely because of glandular disturbances.[46] Psychiatrists routinely reviewed case series of patients with involutional melancholia and reported significantly larger numbers of women than men, and easily explained the numbers with reference to the inevitable and obvious sign of aging in women: menopause.

Physicians in the 1930s increasingly articulated a vision of life as a symmetrical curve—with a rise at the beginning and a decline at the end. In this view, menopause was the mirror image of adolescence. Menopause had been the subject of increasing medical concern by the early twentieth century, and physicians by this time looked to menopause to explain mental and physical problems and to provide a model for treatment.[47] Although not everyone agreed that menopause would result in mental illness, involutional melancholia appeared to be a logical manifestation of a decline in life possibilities and prospects.[48] Physicians did not see the end of productive capacity as the same for men and women, however. Like the climacteric itself, involutional melancholia was thought to be more likely in men in their fifties and sixties, while women were most vulnerable in their forties and fifties. The isolation of ovarian hormones in the 1920s almost immediately led to the use of ovarian hormone preparations for patients with involutional melancholia, but this accelerated even further in the 1930s and 1940s as psychiatrists speculated on the possible endocrine etiology of women's mental disorders.[49]

Menopause provided a clear and convenient marker for mental problems for patients as well as for physicians. In fact, psychiatrists occasionally complained that their patients were too eager to view their emotional problems as directly due to menopause. Clarence Farrar and Ruth MacLachlan Franks of the Toronto Psychiatric Hospital explained in the *American Journal of Psychiatry* in 1931 that many women tended to erroneously assume that they were going to have problems in menopause. Further, physicians were likely to support women in this assumption and treat them accordingly.[50] Farrar and Franks claimed that women would do fine in menopause and that the medical attention to this phase of life for women was overrated, yet their observations about the prevalence of treatment for menopause suggested that they were fighting a losing battle.

Many psychiatrists, convinced of the connection between hormones and mental illness, treated menopausal symptoms and/or involutional melancholia with hormone compounds. These substances, usually provided courtesy of pharmaceutical companies, were available in a variety of forms, including injectible estrogen as well as diethyl stilbestrol (DES).[51] In 1936, a St. Louis University research group studied a group of women with involutional melancholia (which they defined as an extreme version of menopause in which glandular equilibrium was disturbed) by injecting women with a hormonal substance supplied by Park, Davis & Company. This trial bore a number of distinctive characteristics of trials that would be more frequent later in the century: patients were split into treated and control groups, the results were listed by percentage of patients with some degree of improvement (instead of just case study descriptions), and the authors speculated about the benefits of this treatment for the future.[52] Though the research group contained only forty women, the investigators were enthusiastic about the possibilities of hormone therapy for mental illness.

In another published paper from this study, the authors from St. Louis emphasized the importance of involutional melancholia, claiming that 3 to 4 percent of cases of mental illness were due to this ailment. Further, they suggested that menopause itself was on the same spectrum of disease as involutional melancholia. In menopause, "some of these women have the more severe symptoms such as intense subjective nervousness, decreased memory and ability for mental concentration, emotional instability, disturbing mental aberrations and profound depression with thoughts of self-destruction. It is this condition that has been diagnosed as involutional melancholia." Although the team emphasized the severity of the symptoms for their women subjects, they also claimed that their treatment resulted in greater than 90 percent recovery, and boasted that it was safer than the alternatives of the time (including metrazol shock therapy).[53] The researchers published a summary of their studies in the *Journal of the American Medical Association* in 1937 and enthused about the remarkable properties of the hormone preparation, particularly its benefits in restoring productivity to women incapacitated by "physical and mental handicaps."[54] Hormone therapy could be easily administered to outpatients and could theoretically be available to all women, rendering meaningless the distinction between menopause and mental disease.[55]

Not all researchers and clinicians were as enthusiastic about the treatments as the St. Louis University team, but many did pursue the use of hormones in involutional melancholia and were undeterred by negative results. A group in Boston administered hormone preparations to a treatment group of six women and four men, as well as a control group of fourteen women and six men. Although the control group improved and the treatment group did not, the authors of the study were not discouraged by the results, nor did they suggest that this intervention was not worthwhile.[56] A research group from Cornell University tested the effects of the hormone treatments by examining vaginal smears to measure objective effects from the hormone treatments, rather than just using subjective reports of patient improvement. Based on the combination of smears and patient reports, this group found that 5 percent made marked improvement, 30 percent made moderate improvement, while the rest made only slight or no improvement. They concluded that that the treatment did not help severe cases, yet they did not rule out the benefits of the treatment for some.[57] Investigators' strong rationale for giving hormones in involutional melancholia seemed to outweigh their tepid research findings.

Though some researchers did not obtain good results with hormone treatments and criticized their widespread use, clinicians and researchers continued to be attracted by hormone use for involutional melancholia because it brought scientific tools and treatments into psychiatric practice.[58] If involutional melancholia was due to hormone deficits, then animal models could help researchers study the illness.[59] Moreover, new technologies allowed physicians to bring old traditions—such as projecting women's mental disorders onto their bodies—into the future. As psychiatrist Herbert Ripley and pathologist George Papanicolaou (the latter went on to develop the Pap smear) explained, "Since ancient times there has been an appreciation of the fact that menstrual irregularities occur in association with emotional disturbances." The authors buttressed their assertions with slides to demonstrate the connections between mental illness and changes in vaginal smears.[60] In these studies, the Pap smear, which went on to affect the lives of millions of American women, appeared to scientifically link mental problems with hormone changes.[61]

Despite widespread enthusiasm for hormone preparations between the 1920s and the early 1940s, psychiatrists began to shift the focus of their interventions for involutional melancholia to convulsive (or shock) therapies by the late 1940s. Yet the pattern of treatment—particularly the greater number of women in treated groups—continued. As some argued at the time, shock therapies seemed to dramatically improve patients' likelihood of improvement. One psychiatrist examined the prognosis of patients who were treated before the advent of shock treatments (21 men and 40 women) and after the introduction of shock (92 men and 255 women). He found that the patients treated with shock therapies were more likely to have recovered and left the hospital.[62] While the shock therapies were less specific than hormone treatments, they did represent an active treatment that could be done for patients—especially women.

Drastic Times, Drastic Measures

By the 1930s and 1940s, Americans frequently expressed dismay about the state of large psychiatric hospitals, such as the overcrowded conditions and the hopelessness of the inmates there. These difficult conditions fostered and encouraged a variety of what we might consider now to be drastic interventions, particularly convulsive therapies, psychosurgery, and eventually medications.

But the therapies were not evenly applied across all of the hospitalized patient populations. Many of the psychiatrists and neurologists who wrote about patient populations and treatments reported larger numbers of women patients. This is striking since the public hospital census information in 1940 indicated that there were significantly more men in hospitals than women (58 percent men and 42 percent women).[63] Contributors to the medical literature might have noted more women than men in their sample populations by overlooking or dismissing large portions of the hospitalized male patient population, especially those with syphilis, organic brain syndromes, or substance abuse (particularly alcoholism). These diseases did not fill most psychiatrists with enthusiasm about the prospect of treating them.[64]

Instead, physicians' excitement about treatments often correlated with larger numbers of women in their patient populations. For example, in 1948 Paul Huston and Lillian Lochler of the Iowa State Psychopathic Hospital compared manic-depressive patients in a control group of eighty patients (forty-two men and thirty-eight women) with an electroconvulsive therapy (ECT) group of seventy-four patients (twenty-five men and forty-nine women). Although their control group was substantially different, the authors claimed that there was no sex difference in response to the treatment. Further, the authors concluded that their study suggested that shock treatment shortened depression and prevented suicide based on a better outcome for the treated group than the control group.[65] These physicians denied a difference in men's and women's response to treatment, but they did not address the fact that they selected a larger number of women to receive the treatment in the first place. Sex difference was clearly important because it was so carefully noted in studies of somatic treatments.[66] Yet psychiatrists did not appear to find it significant or remarkable that they consistently treated more women than men.

It is possible to read the more aggressive treatment of women as either the result of institutional psychiatric authoritarian practices or psychiatrists' greater propensity to use aggressive therapies to help women.[67] Both of these explanations are compelling. Whether motivated by a desire to help or a desire to control, psychiatrists consistently treated more women than men with specific somatic therapies. Whatever their motives, the preferential treatment of women clearly had an effect on psychiatrists' theories of mental disease. As the pattern of greater treatment of women continued in medication trials, the greater presence of women helped to shape theories about depression, as the treatment defined the disease.

Although there was a clear pattern of higher rates of convulsive therapy treatment of women patients, the medical literature of the time did not explain it.[68] As medications were introduced into psychiatric investigation and practice, physicians continued the older pattern of treating significantly more women than men, but a few did address the rationale of greater medication use in women.[69] Researchers argued (in hindsight) that hospital populations had shifted by the time that medications were introduced. Investigators in the 1960s and 1970s claimed that there had been more older men in hospitals in the pre–World War II era, while by the 1950s and 1960s the hospital population had changed and was comprised of a population of younger, neurotic women. Psychiatrists and others generally claimed that psychiatric treatments of older men had significantly improved (particularly with ECT) such that those men did not need the hospital anymore; therefore, the patients who were in the hospital were those most in need of treatment.[70] (Of course, these observations did not take into account the fact that more women than men had received ECT in the first place.)

Although this account provides insight into researchers' perspectives, it does not match the demographic reality, at least in public hospitals of the time. While the national census data indicated an increase in women patients between 1940 and 1950, only 49 percent of the 1950 psychiatric hospital patients were women. Further, the percentage of women declined again by the 1960 census to 44 percent. What was different about the hospital population during this time period, though, was that psychiatrists significantly shifted how they conceptualized and counted patients by diagnosis. In the 1950 census (as had been the case in 1940), patients were counted by diagnosis and divided into three categories: psychoses (including syphilis, traumatic injuries, involutional psychosis, manic-depressive psychosis, and schizophrenia), psychoneuroses, and mental illness without psychoses (including epilepsy, drug addiction, and alcoholism). Women comprised higher numbers of patients in the psychoneuroses category, as well as some subcategories of psychoses (including schizophrenia), but comprised a significantly smaller portion of the psychoses subcategories of syphilis and alcoholic psychosis. There were also fewer women in the nonpsychotic categories. Because of the ways that patients were classified, it was hard to see a clear pattern relationship between patient diagnosis and sex.[71]

In the 1960 census, however, patients were divided into two main groups—one group that included patients with acute or chronic brain syndromes (in which men predominated) and one group that included patients with psychoses, psychoneuroses, or personality disorders. Women generally predominated in the second group, except that there were more men in the personality disorder subgroup. This kind of division may have produced the impression that the hospital contained a larger group of younger, more neurotic women. The transition in the census categories suggests a conceptual shift in which patients appeared to be divided into those who could be helped (psychotic, psychoneurotic, or personality disordered) and those who could not (brain syndromes).[72]

While the greater number of women in early clinical trials of medications might have had something to do either with more women in hospitals or with the perception that there were more women who could be helped, the number was also partly due to evolving practices of excluding some types of patients from trials. Field studies of emerging medications by the 1960s began to systematically exclude patients with substance abuse from their samples. This had the effect of reducing the number of men who were eligible for studies. Researchers occasionally commented on the possible relationship between alcoholism in particular and depression and suggested that the exclusion of people with alcoholism might skew the numbers. For example, one investigator pointed out in 1971 that the sex differences in prevalence of depression disappeared when male alcoholism was added to female depression in family illness studies.[73] But the evolution of symptom grouping as a way of defining depression made it difficult for researchers to see alcoholism in men as anything related to depression in women.

By the late 1960s and 1970s, medications had shaped the emerging diagnosis of depression within the context of a largely female patient population. Psychiatrists increasingly assumed that women were more vulnerable to depression than men. Yet the data on which researchers made this assumption derived from the settings in which they performed their research. For example, University of Pennsylvania psychiatrist Fritz Freyhan studied a population of depressed patients consisting of 111 women and thirty-six men on a research unit. Freyhan concluded that the sex "ratio of 3:1 corresponds to the sex distribution of admissions, confirming reports in the literature that depression is far more common in women than in men."[74] Depression in women was becoming a circular concept: women were believed to be depressed more than men and were selected for clinical trials more than men, and then their greater presence within trials appeared to affirm that they were depressed more than men.[75] Since it appeared to be self-evident that women suffered from depression more than men, psychiatric researchers shifted their attention toward trying to uncover what specific features in women's biology led them to be more depressed.

Some researchers were so convinced that depression was a disease of women that studies that were done entirely on women were reported as studies on depression itself. For example, the influential Boston–New Haven Collaboration Depression Project, which included such well-known researchers as Myrna Weissman and Gerald Klerman, published extensively on a large-scale study of 150 depressed women, but many of the study's conclusions were explicitly generalized to apply to all patients who were depressed.[76] A few of the papers from this study were published without anything in the title or abstract to indicate that women were the only subjects.[77] This link between women patients and a diagnosis of depression was specific, as research on depressive symptoms on schizophrenia (in which Weissman collaborated) used much larger numbers of men in clinical trials.[78] Further, Weissman and her colleagues designed a form of therapy, known as Interpersonal Psychotherapy (IPT), based on the assumption that depression—as something that happens more in women—was due to disruptions in interpersonal relationships.

Researchers' assumptions about women and their vulnerability to depression were reinforced during the 1970s and 1980s within ongoing shifts in clinical trial methodology. In these years, investigators began to articulate the need to have more homogenous patient populations in order to increase the power of their studies. Indeed, as one reviewer commented in 1976, good research methodology was essential so that practitioners could incorporate the evidence into their clinical decision making: "Clearly, research criteria for patient selection and minimum methodological standards must be adopted before any great amount of clinically useful information can be gleaned from future work in this area."[79] Yet while reviewers were critical of methodological "errors" such as the failure to include an adequate placebo group, researchers' common practice of having significantly more women than men in clinical trials was apparently not noticed.[80]

The sex distribution of those included in clinical trials in psychiatry matters for the conclusions that researchers derived from their studies—even when they could not find statistically significant differences between the ways in which women and men responded to the agents in question. As recently as with the introduction of fluoxetine (Prozac) in the late 1980s, researchers' practice of doing studies on patient populations comprised primarily of women was unchallenged in the psychiatric literature.[81] The pattern of including fewer male subjects in clinical trials on depression could be the reason that the original trials with fluoxetine reported relatively few sexual side effects. The 70 percent of women in the study might not have felt comfortable mentioning sexual side effects. Yet sexual side effects are extremely common in men who receive fluoxetine and other drugs of the same class.[82]

Many current researchers appear to be unaware that women constituted a greater proportion of medication clinical trial subjects over the first decades of antidepressant research, since medical researchers who were exploring other areas at the same time (particularly high blood pressure, diabetes, and high cholesterol) studied primarily (or only) men.[83] In the early 1990s, critics pointed out the scientific problems inherent in evaluating heart disease and its treatment only in men and then generalizing the results to women.[84] Yet the clinical trials of antidepressant medications have not been as critically assessed, despite the fact that the claim that depression is predominantly a women's disease originated in clinical trials that were comprised of mostly (or only) women patients. Further, depression as a disease category was defined around a process of circular reasoning about women. Women were selected for clinical trials because they seemed more depressed (and were not excluded for alcoholism at the same rate as men), which led to counting women's symptoms as those of depression, which led to statistics that show that women are depressed more than men. But despite this shaky logic, the medication-driven experience with depression easily led researchers toward the conclusion that depression must involve some kind of problem in women's biology. While their early-twentieth-century forebears looked at major differences such as menopause, later twentieth-century psychiatrists began to speculate about brain differences.

Researchers in the 1970s worked backward from the presumed effects of antidepressant medications to hypothesize about the mechanism of depression.[85] But at the same time that they were speculating about the effects of neurotransmitters, they also explicitly looked at estrogen on the assumption that the female hormone must have something to do with depression.[86] For example, in 1972 Massachusetts psychiatrist Edward Klaiber and a group set out to measure activity of monoamine oxidase (MAO) in the plasma of depressed patients, based on the observed effects of MAO inhibitors (MAOIs). But they also inquired about estrogen as they specifically examined depressed women, estrogen augmentation, and MAO activity. Though they could not find a relationship between MAO levels and estrogen, Klaiber's group insisted on including hormones as part of the catecholamine hypothesis: "Mental depression is a component of the premenstrual tension syndrome. It is tempting to speculate, therefore, that the premenstrual tension syndrome and psychiatric states of mental depression are two points on a continuum separated by differences in elevation of MAO activity."[87] Klaiber and his group, with some funding from the company that made one of the hormone preparations, gave high-dose estrogen to women patients who had not responded to antidepressant medications. Although the treatment results were not particularly impressive, they were statistically significant, and Klaiber and his group stated that this study justified further work on the role of estrogen in depression.[88]

Although estrogen was the most common hormone studied, researchers occasionally tested other ones. A group in 1974 administered testosterone to five depressed men on the theory that "if being 'more female' worsens the patient's response to imipramine and if being male improves it (as well as lessening the risk for depression), then being 'more male' might further improve the response to imipramine." Instead, the researchers found that four of the men became paranoid. But rather than interpret this as a failure, the group concluded that "it is tempting to say that by using a male hormone we converted the illness of four men from one typical of women to one typical of men."[89] Even in descriptions of depression in men, women's biology and the biology of depression became intertwined in theories about depression and led to further assumptions that depression was a women's disease.[90]

Biological sex differences did not dictate all aspects of research, though. Some investigators were acutely aware that there were social issues that might affect how men and women expressed distress. Psychiatrist and National Institute of Mental Health (NIMH) consultant Dean Schuyler summarized these ideas by pointing out that social mores made it more acceptable for women to talk about their feelings. Further, he suggested that depression might be expressed differently in men and women—and that perhaps alcoholism might be men's usual way of manifesting depression.[91] But though some researchers were cautious about interpreting sex differences in depression, others were much more willing to believe that women not only suffered more from depression but also that the problem was located in women's brains. As psychiatry increasingly embraced the language of science by the 1970s, the scientific "fact" of women's propensity to depression appeared certain, even through the wave of criticism that hit the specialty in the 1970s.

Embracing Diagnoses

Psychiatric theories about women through the post–World War II decades centered on fairly rigid, psychoanalytically inspired ideas about the importance of women for child rearing. Topeka-based psychiatric leader William Menninger provided one of the most sweeping expressions of this idea, arguing that the tremendous number of men rejected for military duty because of psychiatric illness was due to profound problems in American families, including the low birth rate, the increased divorce rate, and the escalating number of women working outside the home.[92] In the worldview of Menninger and others, women's failure to adhere to their gender roles could not only lead to their personal pathology but also to problems in the nation as a whole.

The Cold War–era emphasis on the nuclear family and definitions of domesticity illustrated the ways in which psychological language could be used to interpret and proscribe behavior. While men who were discontented at work could find solace at home, women who were discontented at work (that is, home) went to psychiatrists and psychologists in order to find out how to become better adjusted to that home. The focus of change in this context became the individual, and the psychiatric (or psychological) intervention centered around helping the individual become adapted to the situation rather than changing the situation.[93]

The language of gender roles remained prevalent in the psychiatric literature well into the 1960s and 1970s. While psychiatrists eagerly treated depressed women patients who were passive and helpless, they expressed irritation with needy women who were not satisfied with their home environments.[94] Further, psychiatrists assumed that any domestic unhappiness for women was due to women's unresolved conflicts and unrealistic expectations, particularly of their husbands. For example, one male psychiatrist in 1965 examined the hospital records of fifty physicians' wives who had undergone psychiatric treatment. In his estimation, the women's increasing isolation and despair as their husbands worked long hours were entirely the fault of the women's underlying complexes: "Marriage to an older man, whose vocation may have been unconsciously associated with omnipotent, understanding, protective attributes may be interpreted as an attempt by many of the patients to resolve persisting Oedipal conflicts. Illness developed when the equilibrium of the adjustment was disrupted by such reality factors as the increasing involvement of the doctor in his work, or a conflict between his personality characteristics and the idealized expectations of his wife."[95] According to this author, the answer for these women was for them to resolve their complexes and stop taking their husbands' work schedules personally. At the same time, however, women's self-definition revolved around their relationships to their husbands. Indeed, an individual's conformity to gender expectations was seen as integral to the fabric of society. Women were thus doubly trapped—both by the expectations of restrictive gender roles and by the insistence that any discontent or distress they might feel was entirely an individual pathology.[96]

The implications of psychiatric pronouncements about women were not lost on the emerging feminist movement, and in the 1960s and early 1970s it appeared that there might be an all-out war between feminists and American psychiatrists.[97] In 1963, Betty Friedan outlined the deep sacrifices that women had made to fit the Cold War–era domestic ideology and blamed psychiatrists in particular for suggesting that women were in need of psychiatric treatment when their symptoms resulted from their disempowered position.[98] As the feminist movement accelerated in the 1970s, critiques of women's place within psychiatric pathology proceeded along one of two major lines of argument. One group insisted that misogynist psychiatrists unfairly labeled women as mad or maladjusted. Others argued that the reason so many more women had emotional problems was that social, cultural, economic, and political conditions had been so unfavorable to women that they had no alternatives to madness.[99] Women within the psychiatric profession also pointed to psychiatry's patriarchal past and its ongoing reliance on sexist assumptions.[100] In the 1970s, the American Psychiatric Association's Committee on Women complained to the framers of the third edition of the *Diagnostic and Statistical Manual* (*DSM-III*) that sexist stereotypes about women helped to define the manual's assessment of function.[101] But while feminists in and outside of psychiatry were diligent about calling attention to obvious gender bias, assumptions based on gender continued to permeate theories of health and illness, particularly within the emerging diagnosis of depression.

Depression research proceeded along at a great rate in the 1970s, and researchers and clinicians stated more loudly and more confidently that depression was a disease of women. How did this happen? Researchers did not believe they were unfairly labeling women—in fact, many of them saw the increased attention to depression as part of a greater social movement to pay attention to women's concerns. Some pointed out that depression could be caused by social adversity, including women's often powerless state.[102] While some researchers acted on older assumptions about women's nature and role in society when they described women's depression, others with a more progressive approach also emphasized the importance of treating women for depression.[103] Although all the researchers of this period made assumptions about women consistent with their social and cultural context, a number of them, particularly the prolific Boston-based investigator Myrna Weissman, perceived research on depression to be key to helping women overcome adversity and advance in society.[104]

In fact, depression research helped to create a new dynamic between psychiatrists and women patients, one in which patients' complaints were heard and treated instead of interpreted. While older-style psychiatrists made pronouncements about human behavior based on sexual development, research-based psychiatrists increasingly began to emphasize symptoms. For example, as early as 1959 Washington University researcher George Winkur argued against understanding women patients in terms of unresolved Oedipal conflicts. Instead, "it appears that the best evidence of a psychiatric illness is the presence of a set of specific psychiatric symptoms which are elicited in the usual clinical manner rather than a group of inferences based upon theoretical formulations of etiology and pathogenesis which lead to inappropriate emphasis upon nondiscriminatory phenomena."[105] Winokur's group at Washington University, which would play a leading role in the development of symptom-based psychiatric diagnoses, laid out the issue as a conflict between a psychoanalytic style of imposing an interpretation on a patient and a research style of developing a hypothesis from a set of observations. Many perceived that attention to women's symptoms was a departure from the patriarchal practices of older psychoanalysts.[106]

Researchers' focus on symptoms certainly helped to reduce obvious judgment of women based on gender roles, but the tools with which researchers measured and counted symptoms were themselves affected by gender. These issues are visible through a comparison of symptom rating scales used to monitor depression treatment, particularly differences between the Hamilton Depression Scale (HDS) and the Beck Depression Inventory (BDI). The HDS was developed in Great Britain and published in 1960, and the BDI came out of depression research at the University of Pennsylvania and was published in 1961. These two scales were—and continue to be—widely used as objective measures of the extent of patients' depression. Yet the structure and the content of these scales reflect the social circumstances in which they were constructed.

The HDS, developed by Max Hamilton at the University of Leeds, assessed a variety of symptoms of depression with a particular emphasis on somatic (or physical) symptoms. The scale was designed to be administered by a trained staff person and allowed for both staff observation and patient report of symptoms, including agitation, gastrointestinal symptoms, and other somatic symptoms, as well as hypochondriasis and psychic and somatic anxiety. Only two or three of the items asked patients to respond to a question about how they felt, and there was more emphasis on bodily symptoms than feeling states. The HDS bore little resemblance to the diagnostic category of depression in *DSM-III*, even though the HDS was developed by observing a set of patients and their symptoms. In fact, the reason for the difference is probably that Hamilton designed his scale around a population wholly comprised of male patients.[107]

In contrast to the HDS, which emphasized somatic symptoms and was administered by a professional, the BDI was a self-administered tool that focused more on feeling states.[108] Aaron Beck, the University of Pennsylvania psychiatrist who went on to develop Cognitive Behavioral Therapy (CBT), structured the BDI around a series of questions that asked patients to endorse statements (to varying degrees) about how they felt about themselves and their relationships. There were few items about somatic symptoms in Beck's inventory. Beck's scale was appealing to many who viewed self-assessment scales as less biased than observer scales because they were not subject to investigator interpretation.[109] Beck's scale did look fairly similar to the symptom criteria for depression in the 1970s and the eventual *DSM-III* category of depression, perhaps not a coincidence since his patient population was comprised of close to 70 percent women.

Both the BDI and the HDS were used in the United States in the decades after their introduction, and both allowed researchers to track items affected by the treatment that was being studied. Hamilton's scale focused on physiological signs and symptoms that were likely to be produced by antidepressants that were being tested at the time, while Beck's scale effectively tracked patients' improvement with his structured therapy, CBT.[110] But though these assessment instruments were intended to provide objective, measurable indications of patients' depression, most researchers appeared unaware or unconcerned about the ways in which the assessment tool design affected their outcomes—particularly around issues of gender. Hamilton went back and reassessed his rating scale in 1967 and determined that women scored differently in some areas, but researchers in the 1960s and 1970s frequently used the HDS to measure drug effects without attention to possible differences between men and women in scoring this scale.[111] In addition, the large number of somatic symptoms incorporated in the HDS did not seem to influence researchers who translated their clinical experience with patients and medications into diagnostic criteria. Further, even though Beck's group found in 1974 that the BDI diagnosis of depression correlated strongly with female sex in screening populations, they concluded that this in fact represented a true measure of depression.[112] Researchers and epidemiologists who used Beck's scale did not address the issue of how men might respond to a screening tool that asked multiple questions about how they felt about themselves—even though, as historians of masculinity have pointed out, American men since the mid-twentieth century have faced strong cultural taboos against expressing feelings.[113]

The diagnostic criteria that emerged for depression in the 1970s were also strongly influenced by the patient populations in which they were developed and the assumptions of the researchers. And, like the rating scales, they appeared to select for symptoms that would be experienced more by women.

John Feighner and his group at Washington University, the authors of the first diagnostic criteria paper from 1972, devised their criteria for depression in the context of their ongoing studies of depression. In a study population from the same year as their diagnostic criteria paper, the Washington University group had forty-nine patients, sixteen men and thirty-three women, a distribution they explained by saying that the "overall group characteristics showed similarity to the age range and sex ratio typical of primary depressions." Of course, Feighner and his group had already excluded patients with other diagnoses, including alcoholism. (Incidentally, this study, which unsuccessfully attempted hormone augmentation to supplement treatment of depressed patients with imipramine or ECT, was criticized by a commentator who said that the hormone therapy would have been shown to be effective if the researchers had not included so many men in the study.)[114] In order to define research criteria for depression, Feighner and his group counted all of the symptoms of the patients they thought were depressed and then selected the symptoms that were most consistent across the group. The criteria for depression the researchers used, which were published in a slightly different form in their nomenclature paper, became the core symptoms that would be expanded by others, including Robert Spitzer and his colleagues at the New York State Psychiatric Institute, to form the diagnosis of depression in the third and subsequent editions of *DSM*.[115] While Feighner's group devised the depression criteria in order to have a consistent basis for patient selection in clinical trials, they also clearly had an expectation of what their treatment population would look like as they excluded those who had complicating factors such as alcoholism.

Like Feighner and his colleagues, Spitzer was also motivated to have criteria that generated patient groups about which there would be little professional disagreement.[116] But the New York researcher's contribution was primarily to loosen the restrictions of the diagnosis and to include more symptom possibilities (and thus more patients).[117] The transition from Spitzer's Research Diagnostic Criteria (RDC) to *DSM-III* criteria further lowered the threshold for diagnosis.[118] The clustering together of patients with particular symptoms definitely produced more agreement, but did it represent diagnosis, or was it more a representation of how researchers perceived patients? Further, the fewer and fewer symptoms and shorter time period required to make the diagnosis of depression helped to validate more patient concerns, but the lowered threshold also enormously expanded the number of people who could be described as depressed—a majority of them women.

In these foundation studies for the diagnosis of depression, researchers gathered together a group of patients who qualified for their idea of depression (after excluding patients with substance abuse), counted up all of these patients' symptoms, and then listed the most common symptoms as the criteria for depression. This diagnostic criteria design is remarkably circular—patients were defined as depressed because they matched researchers' assumptions about what depression looked like (often because they responded to medication that seemed to help with depression), and their symptoms were used to diagnose depression in general. The researchers explicitly excluded substance-abusing patients and included those who could articulate symptoms of depression. Most of the diagnosis, then, rested on patients' subjective impressions of their troubles and psychiatrists' assumptions about what to do about them.

The criteria for depression published in *DSM-III*—criteria developed through clinicians' experiences with largely female patient populations—were directly translated into population data through the Epidemiologic Catchment Area (ECA) study in the early 1980s.[119] In the ECA study, as well as others since that time, the diagnosis of depression was not only used without question but also was used to screen the population for the presence of depression. Researchers and epidemiologists assumed that it was valid to use criteria that had been determined in a hospitalized population in order to test the public for untreated or undiagnosed illness.[120] Further, the ECA and other epidemiological researchers used survey instruments that focused on individual endorsement of feeling states. For example, one of the most commonly used screening tools was the Center for Epidemiologic Studies Depression Scale (CES-D), a self-rating scale of twenty items, over half of which asked people to assess their feelings about themselves.[121] Perhaps not surprisingly, when researchers asked men and women about their feeling states, more women than men endorsed feeling depressed. Further, when epidemiological researchers used the criteria for depression in the general population (criteria that had been developed in a patient population that was generally two-thirds or more women), they found that more women than men endorsed the symptoms (at a ratio of about two to one).

Two important aspects of depression research in the 1970s and 1980s reinforced psychiatrists' conviction that depression was primarily a women's disease. First, researchers sought out ways to make their clinical trial samples of patients as homogenous as possible and often focused exclusively on women patients in order to reduce variation in the patient population.[122] Second, researchers eliminated features of the depression diagnosis that might have included more men. One of the significant features that current psychiatrists see in depressed men is irritability, but this mood descriptor was eliminated from the diagnosis of depression by *DSM-IIIR* (published in 1987).[123]

While it might be tempting to view the process of describing the diagnosis of depression in women as pathologizing experiences more common in women, psychiatrists have appeared to be motivated primarily by their conviction that women were suffering and needed their help.[124] For example, a group from the University of Hawaii studied the wives of navy submarine personnel and found that these women developed "clinical levels of depression" during their husbands' absences. The authors were clearly invested in helping these women and published an appeal from one woman who wanted the navy to stop the difficult three-month on, three-month off submarine rotations—if only to benefit the wives, whatever the effect on their husbands.[125] Whether or not the women patients who were part of the depression studies in the 1970s and 1980s felt validated in these studies, researchers perceived that their endeavors were necessary in order to help widespread suffering—especially in women.

Further, the profession's particular attention to depression in women evolved at the same time that increasing numbers of women entered psychiatry.[126] Women psychiatrists in the late 1970s and 1980s often articulated their interest in helping women patients. Some of the early women leaders of the field, keenly aware of the challenges of working and raising families, suggested that women's complicated social roles made them vulnerable to depression. Further, some women researchers' personal experiences and the experiences of other women physicians made them more sympathetic to women's emotional difficulties.[127] From these perspectives, attention to depression in women reflected professional interest in the welfare of women patients from male—and increasingly female—psychiatrists.[128]

But in the meantime, what about men? While crises of work had propelled men toward neurologists' offices (and sometimes psychiatric institutions) in the early part of the century, prevailing ideals of masculinity by the decades after World War II left little room for psychological problems. While men might have felt trapped by the imperative of work productivity, particularly the potential conflict between aspiring to masculine standards and avoiding faceless conformity, they did not necessarily go to psychiatrists for such problems.[129] Some men's struggles with gender roles were the subject of psychiatric interest—especially around the issue of homosexuality. Still, psychiatrists after World War II seemed much less enthusiastic about interpreting men's discontent as mental illness.[130] Men's distress—to the extent that it was described at all by psychiatrists—was left out of the emerging diagnosis of depression in the second half of the century.

The virtual silence on depression in men in medical literature through the 1990s did not mean a lack of research on mental problems in men, however, as investigators did explore issues of substance abuse.[131] While several researchers emphasized that men who had substance abuse problems might well be displaying symptoms of depression, other investigators came to different conclusions. For example, one group at a Veterans' Administration facility in South Carolina studied different rating scales applied to recently detoxified alcoholic men and found that the rates of measured depression depended on the rating scales used: 28 percent screened positive with the HDS, 66 percent screened positive with an assessment tool called the Zung Depression scale (similar to the BDI), and 43 percent screened positive with the Minnesota Multiphasic Personality Inventory (MMPI).[132] In contrast to these large numbers, clinical interviews only revealed about 9 percent depression among the men in the study. Although rating scales, with their emphasis on context-free symptoms, were often used in other studies to uncover cases of depression in women, these researchers argued against this approach for men. Instead, the South Carolina study authors concluded that alcoholic men should be interviewed (rather than rated) because the rating scales would lead to inappropriate diagnosis and treatment for depression.[133] Further, researchers at the University of Washington in Seattle studied medication effects in recovering alcoholic men and argued that symptom relief came at the expense of the ability to function in rehabilitation.[134] Clearly, the conclusions researchers derived from their clinical studies of men and women depended on their expectations and their assumptions about gender and mental illness.[135]

In asserting that mental diseases were best categorized by symptoms (particularly in women), researchers in the twentieth century took phenomena that were shaped by social, cultural, economic, and gender factors and made them the basis for diagnosis of mental illness.[136] It is not surprising that the diagnosis of depression reflects the social, cultural, and gender contexts of its emergence in the 1970s and 1980s. It is worrisome, therefore, that a diagnosis of depression that is so historically contingent should be the basis of ongoing research that looks at differences between brains of men and women in order to uncover the biochemical basis of this disease. But it is also a concern that disease diagnosis has become so important in validating individuals' (especially women's) distress.

Although feminists and others concerned about some psychiatric diagnoses (especially personality disorders and premenstrual disorders) have accused psychiatrists of labeling normal variants of behavior as disease, most women do not perceive psychiatrists to be exerting power through labels. As the culture of psychiatric practice moved beyond late-nineteenth- and early-twentieth-century coercive institutional practices, and past twentieth-century psychoanalytic value judgments, psychiatrists began to exercise power through persuasion and validation. Late-twentieth-century and early-twenty-first century women have bought into the idea that symptoms such as low mood, changes in sleep and appetite, decreased interest or motivation, and feelings of hopelessness represent a disease. Many women seek out a diagnosis because it suggests that their problems are caused by an agent outside of their control and that they can be treated through medications. Psychiatrists do not need to tell anyone that they are sick—most psychiatric practices are crowded with patients, and psychiatrists do not need to recruit. Instead, psychiatric power now is located in the definition of distress as a disease through which physicians validate patients' distress and offer them treatment.[137] Women have been avid consumers of this way of conceptualizing and treating their feelings.

Throughout the years of defending their specific psychiatric diagnoses, New York State Psychiatric Institute researcher Robert Spitzer and his colleagues addressed a number of challenges to diagnostic criteria based on concerns about gender bias. Although those who have accused the *DSM* framers of gender bias argue that psychiatrists pathologize women, defenders of the system insist that they have been making appropriate scientific observations (based on available data) and helping patients in need. The conflicts between these two positions have been quite heated and have taken place inside and outside the psychiatric literature, as well as inside and outside the convention halls where the American Psychiatric Association (APA) has met.[138]

One of the major critiques made about some diagnostic categories is that they punish women for acting in gender-specific ways. For example, psychologist Pamela Reed Gibson has pointed out that the *DSM* diagnostic category of histrionic personality disorder, a disorder characterized by "excessive emotionality and attention seeking," is laden with pitfalls in its construction and its diagnosis around women's expressions of distress.[139] She argues that the concept of "hysterical" is applied "about women when they seek help and make the mistake of showing strong emotion to a clinical observer."[140] Women have the social and cultural role of expressing feelings, yet if they are too emotional or too aggressive in their expression of emotions, they are at risk to be diagnosed with a personality disorder.

Critics of Premenstrual Dysphoric Disorder (PMDD), the diagnosis that involves mental symptoms connected to women's menstrual function, have also argued that it is not fair to diagnose large numbers of women in the context of their regular physiology. As psychologist Paula Caplan has pointedly asked, "Do half a million American women go crazy once a month?"[141] Caplan described the political process through which the diagnosis of PMDD achieved its current legitimacy (it is technically in the appendix of *DSM-IV-TR*, but can be diagnosed and treated—and billed for) and has pointed out the political—and contingent—process through which the category was accepted by the APA. Although PMDD has specific criteria and is not intended to be used for all women, it harkens back to centuries of physicians' assumptions about the potentially harmful role of women's reproductive systems.[142]

The same arguments against PMDD and personality disorders could be made against depression—researchers and clinicians blame physiological function for the generation of mental disease, and psychiatric characterizations of women (especially their social connectedness) are used both to describe women and to explain their vulnerability to disease.[143] But advocates of women's mental health—even those with a stated feminist agenda—argue that women benefit from more aggressive diagnosis and treatment of disorders, like depression, that are more prevalent in women. Epidemiologists have asserted that depression is significantly more common in women than in men, while psychopharmacologists have explored the differences in medication response for men and women.[144] Many of the researchers who work in the area of gender differences in mood disorders argue that women deserve to have their mental experiences validated, and that appropriate recognition and treatment of mental disorders in women are part of an agenda for equal rights for women in medicine.

There has not been much feminist—or other kind—of protest against the diagnosis of depression, nor have there been heated claims about gender bias in this diagnosis.[145] In the last several decades, it has made a fair amount of sense for both psychiatrists and the public to see depression in terms of something that typically happens to women for both biological and social reasons.[146] But what exactly is the evidence that depression is more common in women? There does seem to be evidence that depressive symptoms—particularly as they are measured and counted now—are more common in women. But what is the relationship between symptoms and disease? There has been some suggestion that symptoms are different within specific populations, such as the elderly.[147] Do men and women experience the same kinds of symptoms?[148] What about other factors such as class, race, and living situation?[149]

The issue with depression is clearly more than psychiatrists' propensity to see pathology in women. Instead, it suggests that the gender assumptions that were operative at the construction of the diagnosis of depression affected who would be diagnosed. In 1967, University of Michigan researcher Monica Blumenthal found that men and women responded differently to questions about mental symptoms, and that their responses had different relationships to the likelihood of diagnosis of mental illness.[150] Further, as some health behavioral analysts pointed out in the early 1980s, obtaining psychiatric help required three steps: identifying something as a problem, deciding that the problem needed treatment, and getting connected with resources to help with that problem. In their analysis, women were much more likely than men to translate their experiences into problems. Thus the sex bias that these authors uncovered took place on the level of the patient's willingness or ability to name an experience as a problem.[151] All of these researchers postulated that men and women had different social roles and that men were socialized to be less willing to identify their experiences as evidence of mental disease. Although social roles for men and women have loosened considerably in the decades since these studies were published, there is likely still a gender gap in symptom identification.

Not only might male and female patients experience distress differently, but also there remains a question of whether men and women might enact illness behavior in different ways. Some have in fact suggested that men might be more likely to abuse substances while women might be more likely to become depressed—each seeks a medication, but in different forms. Although this has been a frequent observation in the literature, it does not seem to have affected the ways in which either depression or substance abuse diagnoses have been formulated. One issue is that the literature on substance abuse has little connection with the literature on depression. Do men who manifest substance abuse symptoms have a similar biochemical problem as women with depression but their disease course looks different?[152] Or do they have the same symptoms or internal experiences as women but use substances in response? Further, should men who develop depressive symptoms and have alcohol problems be treated as depressed or as alcoholic?[153] And how will these reported differences between men and women change as men's and women's social and cultural roles continue to change over time?

Although the constructed nature of the depression diagnosis raises major issues about psychiatrists' diagnostic and treatment patterns, a critique of depression from only the perspective of psychiatrists misses the powerful draw that the disease category of depression has had among American women. Many women have become invested in framing their problems as depression—a disease for which they can seek treatment. This diagnosis does not work as well for men, though; for many men, there continues to be a disconnect between masculine ideals and depressive symptoms. Psychiatrists generally mean well and want to help their patients—and they have created a category of illness that captures an enormous range of feelings and behavior in women. But are all of these feelings and behavior part of a disease process?[154]

The new power of psychiatry—that of offering an external solution to problems of low mood, low energy, hopelessness, and fluctuations in appetite and sleep—is that it takes the blame (and the responsibility) away from the individual who is suffering. While a medical model of depression still locates the problem within the individual who needs to be fixed, the solution to the problem does not have to come from within the individual. Modern psychiatry, therefore, is not as much coercive as it is persuasive. Its appeal to patients dovetails nicely with the pharmaceutical companies' efforts to get patients to want medications for their problems. Nevertheless, the consumer desire for depression treatments that has been tapped by the pharmaceutical industry significantly predated the industry's direct marketing efforts. Not only psychiatrists but also the public have seen depression as a problem for women.

Chapter 5

Feelings and Relationships

In late July 1972, Senator Thomas Eagleton withdrew his candidacy for vice president on George McGovern's Democratic ticket only days after his selection because of controversy over his revelation that he had been treated for "nervous exhaustion" in the 1960s.[1] Some of Eagleton's colleagues in Washington, D.C., reported that this was not news to them, and that it was common knowledge among politicians that Eagleton was a "high-strung guy."[2] But while some of Eagleton's political colleagues had been aware of his history, McGovern evidently had not. Although Eagleton received a fair amount of public and political support after the news of his history of psychiatric treatment, McGovern did not believe that Eagleton would be an asset to the ticket.[3] After several days of intense media coverage on the issue, Eagleton withdrew from the race, apparently at McGovern's request.[4] Many had expressed their admiration of Eagleton for overcoming his emotional problems, but political decision makers and some of the public thought that Eagleton's future emotional stability could not be assured with the stress of public office.[5]

Eagleton's revelation came at a time of transition of popular accounts of mental illness, from nervousness to anxiety to depression.[6] Further, the media frenzy around Eagleton's disclosure illustrated that mental illness was connected to gender roles. By the 1970s and 1980s, much of the popular discussion around mood and depression centered on internal feelings—but primarily for women. The public was clearly uncomfortable with the idea that a male politician was subject to his feelings. In addition, depression narratives increasingly began to focus on intimate relationships. Eagleton's story, though, did not mention any intimate relationships—instead, his illness and treatment were exposed in the context of a contentious political process. Finally, popular discussions about mental illness over the century increasingly focused on the power and necessity of consumption to solve emotional problems. With this shift, Eagleton's history of having received electroconvulsive therapy (ECT) raised the question of his ability to take control as a man.[7]

Eagleton's story illustrates the poor fit between men's depression and the growing public understanding of the illness. While early-twentieth-century popular literature had described nervous men as well as nervous women, depression stories in the second half of the century strongly emphasized women's experiences. Indeed, popular magazines directed primarily at women not only focused women's attention on the problem of depression but also led the way for other popular magazine portrayals of mood problems. While the medical press highlighted women's symptoms, especially their feelings, popular magazines helped to create a context for those symptoms by encouraging emotional expression and the expectation that everyone should be happy. Depression emerged as a quintessential women's phenomenon as it seemed to highlight women's issues, particularly the role of feelings, the importance of intimate relationships, and the power of consumption to solve problems.[8] Popular magazine writers accepted what appeared to be a growing consensus that women comprised the majority of depression's victims and reinforced connections between women's attributes and the diagnosis. Women did not protest the higher rates of depression because it seemed to capture women's struggles during decades when they faced the paradoxes of greater freedoms and more responsibilities at home and at work.

Depression had become so thoroughly enmeshed within popular discussions of women's expectations and circumstances that descriptions of depression in men, including Eagleton's and other men's descriptions that were more common by the early 1990s, sounded different and strange. Indeed, while popular commentators mentioned the risk of stigma in depression diagnosis, the only places where stigma appeared to be a major issue was around the diagnosis of men's depression.[9] By 1990, depression appeared to be part of a range of normal female responses to stresses in relationships. Even without citing numbers and statistics, American popular literature clearly illustrated that depression was a woman's disease.

The Role of Feelings

Depression's definition now relies on patient endorsement of a number of (presumably) abnormal feeling states. Researchers who defined the depression diagnostic criteria took for granted that all potential or actual patients shared a common vocabulary about feelings and could articulate problematic ones. But is there a shared vocabulary of feelings? And does it change over time? Although popular magazines cannot illustrate all of American understandings about feelings, they can document change over time and the evolution of specific differences in the vocabulary of feelings for men and women.

In the early twentieth century, most popular magazine descriptions of nervousness postulated some kind of external cause for symptoms for women as well as for men. For example, modern civilization appeared to be taking a toll on women because of their sensitive, emotional natures. As the Reverend Samuel McComb of the popular Boston Emmanuel Movement explained, "women's nervous organization is finer and more delicate than man's: the keen edge of a razor is more easily turned than the blunt iron of an axe."[10] While women were overly sensitive all the time, commentators explained that men could become sensitive through overwork and failure to engage in appropriate leisure.[11] For both women and men, the solution was to learn to manage feelings—women by not overindulging them, men by subsuming them into active pursuits. Feelings were not the cause of the problem, but rather something to be managed to solve the problem.

For women, having exquisitely sensitive feelings was not necessarily a good thing. Physician John Mitchell complained in 1901 that "there are plenty of women who think it feminine and interesting to be in a continual sizzle of excitement about little matters, and who thus acquire not only false standards of feeling, but presently a total inability to feel genuinely or simply about anything."[12] According to many commentators, while women might be under the impression that indulging in excessive feelings was feminine, in fact women were too selfish and self-absorbed if they were overly tuned in to their own emotional states.

Excessive indulgence in feelings was a major risk for nervous men, too. Popular authors exhorted men to seek out activities that would strengthen their masculinity, not increase their likelihood of becoming prostrate with feelings. As one author suggested, reading was an appropriate diversion for neurotic men, but it had to be the right kind: "If the neurotic can get hold of literature that is 'strong' because it is virile and not because it is vile, he will be giving his mind a first class medicine."[13] Men needed appropriately masculine pursuits outside work, but they also needed to avoid being overly emotional.[14] Excessive emotional indulgence, particularly at work, might make men angry and frustrated with others or even tearful, and potentially decrease their work efficiency.

For both men and women in the first half of the century, the tumultuous changes of modern life increased the peril of excessive emotional expression, and authors of popular advice encouraged men and women to carefully manage their feelings. It was not until the second half of the century, when language of psychological conflicts and an emotional inner life permeated much of American society, that emotional expression became a part of identity.[15] Yet men and women did not have equal opportunities for this expression, as the narrowing of masculine definitions placed feelings within the sole purview of women.

In the second half of the century, many popular magazines—especially women's magazines—began to take on more of a role of providing advice. As written periodicals attempted to compete in an entertainment market that increasingly included other formats such as television, magazine editors solicited articles on information and advice topics, including mental illness and emotional distress.[16] Women's magazines in particular emphasized the risks, benefits, trials, and tribulations of individual efforts to manage feelings. In these popular discussions of emotions, depression was a feeling, a mood, a state of mind, and sometimes a disease. But no matter how commentators explained it, they encouraged their women readers to understand, to talk about, and to deal with their feelings.

The first major popular magazine accounts of depression in the late 1950s and 1960s stressed the role of women's feelings and the importance of validating them. These initial articles described the phenomenon of sadness in the days after childbirth and the challenges to women of adjusting to life with a baby. Authors, often physicians or journalists who interviewed physicians, described typical cases of women who felt bad and explained why they might feel this way.[17] In 1967, Indiana University obstetrician Sprague Gardner stressed the value of education about feelings: "The woman who knows that after-birth blues are a natural occurrence, an experience shared by most new mothers, can prepare in advance to meet the situation intelligently. She can be alert for the feeling, recognize it as part of the continuing process of childbirth and anticipate its passing."[18] Women's magazines over the next few decades emphasized not only that women could and would feel strong emotions at different times, but also that women's feelings were important and worthy of discussion.[19]

The messages about depression spread outward from the women's magazines toward other audiences. Just as the markets for products originally intended for adults crept into the emerging magazine market for teenage girls, depression descriptions also made an increasing appearance in teenager-directed magazines.[20] Teen magazines offered advice and self-help tips as writers explained to female readers that they could experience the same emotional problems as their mothers, teachers, and grandmothers.[21] Within the broad range of emotions freely discussed in teen magazines, it was not clear whether depression represented a normal teenage problem or a major catastrophe. But whether writers encouraged teenagers to accept their feelings as normal or to take action, what was at stake was girls' growing responsibility regarding emotional expression.[22] Teenage girls needed to be able to speak the language of feelings, including the language of depression.

Throughout popular magazine descriptions of depression, particularly in women's magazines, writers coupled their descriptions of feelings with exhortations to readers to take action. At the same time that feelings, including depressive ones, appeared to be normal for women, it did not mean that they should be accepted. As New York physician Helen DeRosis argued in an article for *Harper's Bazaar*, depression was a maladaptive coping mechanism for women: "Avoid using depression as a way of coping when problems occur, for a mild depression can escalate into a severe one. And depression can be addictive—for if you don't learn to prevent it now, you may have these debilitating up-and-down periods throughout the rest of your life."[23] DeRosis and her coauthor, Victoria Pellegrino, ran workshops for women in New York to help them fight back against the symptoms of depression.[24]

One of the ways that women learned they could fight bad feelings was through exercise. Journalists reported that researchers found that physical exercise was as effective as medications or psychotherapy for mild to moderate depression.[25] But beyond that, exercise provided a way for women to gain control of their bodies, a task that appeared increasingly important in magazines that focused on women's homes and in those that emphasized their political equality.[26] In addition, most of the advice literature acknowledged that exercise while feeling depressed was quite difficult—women who could pull it off were demonstrating the admirable quality of self-control.[27]

Writers often used the same language of self-improvement to describe overcoming depression that they used to explain weight loss. Indeed, by 1990 accepting a bad mood in women's magazines was as unthinkable as accepting obesity.[28] And as they did with issues of weight, writers increasingly argued that women were not destined for a particular mental state but could change themselves. As a *Mademoiselle* writer explained in 1990 in an article entitled "Smile: The Mood Makeover," "We're raised to suffer through bouts of the blues as if they're a strain of the flu: inexorable, unstoppable and impossible to resist. But actually, a sad attitude, unlike the common cold, is something you can control, take charge of and change . . . it all begins with realizing the options at your disposal, then trying serious strategies to lift your spirits."[29] For women's magazines, the common cold metaphor for depression worked, not only to reassure women that depression was common but also to empower them to cure themselves. Women's fluency in the language of feelings translated into constant strivings for internal—as well as external—perfection.

Though women in the second half of the century were strongly encouraged not only to feel but also to take charge of their feelings, men in American society had diminishing emotional options during this time period. The model of masculinity, first articulated in the 1950s, that affected most of the popular discussion of depression in men was one of detachment and stoicism. Within this model, men could not (nor should they) express feelings about anything, never mind sadness. Not surprisingly, John Wayne, the infamous symbol of aggressive masculinity throughout the middle of the century, denied that he ever had periods of feeling down when asked (along with other celebrities) in 1976.[30] Accounts of depression in women's magazines had blurred the line between feelings and depression, but men's experiences were different. When men did have feelings, those feelings were completely overwhelming and impossible to manage. In 1969, an *Esquire* writer described British politician Winston Churchill's battle with his "black dog" depression.[31] News correspondent Percy Knauth published an account in 1972 of his own battle with depression, and described how foreign this experience was to his normal activities as a man.[32] Writer William Styron, in his book *Darkness*, expressed his experience with depression in terms of something that took control of him. As a *People* article described in 1990, Styron's book "stresses the crucial difference between everyday blues, which we also blithely call depression, and the blanketing darkness that transforms all pleasures into 'indistinguishable ordeals of fogbound horror.'"[33] The language of feelings that was so critical in describing women's depression in this time period—particularly identifying problematic feelings and taking action to deal with them—did not work for men's depression. Men who became depressed were completely incapacitated and unable to articulate or manage their feelings.

While women discovered things about themselves through introspection, mood problems in men almost always seemed to connect to external events or conflicts, especially around work.[34] According to observers, men's problems originated from the constriction of men's work opportunities in the 1970s and 1980s. The economy, not the individual, could be blamed for men's depression.[35] Journalist Ellen Goodman said in a *McCall's* article that she had observed that more men of her acquaintance became depressed because their expectations to achieve greatness were more likely to be disappointed than women's already lower expectations.[36] A few men in competitive sports became depressed because of the stress under which they were working—which subsequently caused a "chemical imbalance."[37] Some American farmers appeared to be at risk because of the increasing financial troubles inherent in 1980s farming.[38] Indeed, financial problems in a variety of occupations could lead to increased depression in men, even in those who had been moderately, or even greatly, successful.[39] Thus for men, depression arose from struggle in the modern world against the increasing onslaught of modern, impersonal bureaucracy—rather than a problem with feelings.[40]

While early-twentieth-century accounts of nervousness identified overindulgence in feelings as a problem for both men and women, popular magazine discussions of depression in the second half of the century appeared to set no limit to the amount of feelings women could or should express. Descriptions of depression by and about women emphasized introspection as key to identifying and dealing with depression. For men, however, feelings could be a catastrophe, particularly if they interfered with work. While early-twentieth-century men had the opportunity for at least some feelings (as long as they were not overly indulged), masculine ideals in the later part of the century suggested that emotional expression in men was highly suspect.[41]

Relationships

At the same time that popular magazines illustrated shifts in appropriate expressions of feelings, particularly the differences between men and women by the second half of the twentieth century, they also illustrated change with regard to relationships. In the first half of the century, popular commentators did not usually incorporate discussions of intimate relationships in their descriptions of either nervous disease or insanity. Yet in the second half of the century, intimate relationships achieved center stage with the emerging discussions of depression, especially in women's magazines. Writers insisted that relationships were more important to women, and that disruptions in these relationships would lead to depression. Men did not appear to be equal partners, though, as women carried the responsibility for emotional matters. Over the span of the century, mental illness (nervousness and insanity) moved inward, from its origins in society to its origins within internal experience structured by close relationships. In this area, as in others, women appeared more vulnerable.

In the early decades of the twentieth century, nervousness (as well as insanity) in both men and women appeared in the context of broad social changes for both sexes. Commentators articulated their views—both positive and negative—about the increasing roles of women in public life, while men's context was their work life. Neither popular writers nor physicians appeared to think that nervousness was caused by problems in close relationships, and in fact relationships were not mentioned as precipitating circumstances in popular explanations of nervous problems. Instead, nervousness was a manifestation of the shifting social environment that challenged early-twentieth-century men and women.

At a time when women increasingly argued about expanding their social and political spheres, commentators often used the presence of nervous diseases in women to point the finger at what they considered to be inappropriate extensions of women's roles.[42] As Boston Psychopathic Hospital psychiatrist Abraham Myerson wrote in the *Ladies' Home Journal* in 1920, nervousness in society was directly due to women's ambition: "The neurosis of the housewife has a large part of its origin in the increasing desires of women, in their demands for a fuller more varied life than that afforded by the lot of the housewife. Dissatisfaction, discontent, disgust, discouragement, hidden or open, are part of the factors of the disease."[43] But though individual women might express discontent with their particular situation, the problem was clearly a broad social one in which a mismatch had occurred between more traditional and modern activities for women.

Although Myerson was more descriptive than judgmental, others were harshly critical of women's desires outside the home. In 1912, Max Schlapp, identified as a neuropathologist at Cornell University, expounded on the dangers to civilization from changes in women's activities. In Schlapp's view, women's diversion of their nervous energies toward work perverted their offspring: "When overwrought women have disturbed within themselves the processes of nature, they impart a disturbance to their offspring, and, as in the case of fish, instead of the development of a normal human being, there is one distorted in body or mind, or in both. It is fundamental that the female must be quiescent."[44] Schlapp particularly targeted women's dangerous activities such as demanding equal rights with men, and argued that women needed to return to the home and motherhood in order to rescue modern civilization.[45]

While women's efforts at emancipation represented both an individual and a social problem, men's activities could also be dangerous since irrational thinking might lead to dangerous political problems. In 1923, Dr. Stewart Paton explained that psychoneuroses were more dangerous than insanity because their rise "explains the vogue of certain movements and cults that appear absurd and ridiculous to the normal person."[46] Of course, labeling political ideas as products of mental or nervous disturbance indicated that the boundary between normal and pathological behavior in men was not only a matter of hygiene but also a matter of national security.[47] For both men and women, mental pathology represented as much a social as an individual problem.

While women's and men's social worlds shaped popular magazine descriptions of nervousness in the first half of the century, the context of mental distress shifted after World War II. The nuclear family achieved a new significance in American life as both context and cause of emotional distress.[48] Men and women clearly had different levels of investment in the nuclear family, as men spent much of their time in their own work environments. Women therefore became identified as being responsible for happiness in the home. As popular magazine commentators indicated, this made them more vulnerable to depression because of disruptions in intimate relationships, but it also put them in the position of being guardians of the family's emotional health. While some women complained about the confines of domestic ideology, few women complained about the perception that women were the emotional centers of their families.[49]

As women's social world began to change by the 1960s and 1970s, writers continued to emphasize the importance of individual women's adjustment to those changes. Instead of suggesting that society's expectations—that women retain their 1950s-style domestic obligations while grudgingly allowing them to work full time—were unfair or unrealistic, writers put the focus on individual women and their ability to cope.[50] Some writers described women's depression in the 1970s and 1980s as the consequence of their overloaded expectations and schedules.[51] Others pointed out that women's expectations about their lives had been disappointed, since social changes had not relieved their burdens at home.[52] For African American women, as psychoanalyst Marie Saunders suggested in *Essence* in 1980, depression was directly the result of the double oppression of racial and gender discrimination. As women struggled against enormous forces holding them back, it was natural that they should become depressed.[53] But as a 1986 *Essence* article suggested, African American women particularly needed to fight against depression not only to combat the feelings but also the reality of ongoing social problems and the perception by many that therapy was only for white people.[54] Regardless of their political stance, these accounts all assumed that greater opportunities for women and increased oppression could cause individual women to become depressed—and that the answer was to treat individual women.

Despite the perception that women had new choices and opportunities that they never had before—or perhaps because of it—commentators emphasized the ways in which women were likely to suffer from depression due to conflicts within their intimate relationships. Throughout the decades, women's connection to others was reiterated again and again by women, in women's magazines, and in general readership periodicals. Women's ability to get close to others was cited as a reason for women's increased rate of depression, but this was also women's strength in that they could fully engage in supportive and meaningful relationships.

Journalist Maggie Scarf became one of the most vocal and active proponents of the idea that women's depression related to their relationships with others, as outlined in her best-selling and somewhat controversial book, *Unfinished Business*, in 1980.[55] Scarf interviewed a large number of women to find out what their depressions had in common. She discovered that women had a higher investment in relationships with others, and that because of disruptions in these relationships, women were more likely to become depressed.[56] Although Scarf worried about the prevalence of depression in women, she celebrated women's capacities to engage in meaningful, intimate relationships.

Scarf's views about women's essential differences from men, described during the height of the feminist movement, were certainly not accepted without question.[57] Yet Scarf was widely cited and was able to explain why women, even those who were actively pursuing careers, appeared more vulnerable than men to depression.[58] At the same time that feminist historians were making important observations about women's social networks of the past, Scarf's observations about women's need for continued social networks seemed to make sense.[59] Indeed, some were able to explain women's greater capacity to achieve social connectedness as both a risk factor and a treatment for depression.[60]

But though intimate relationships shaped the context and the importance of women's depression, commentators by no means suggested that women seek liberation from these relationships. Instead, activists argued that women should use the empowerment they gained from other aspects of their lives to overcome depression. As psychologist Harriet Braiker explained in *Working Woman* in 1987, a woman who responded to depression at home by becoming passive and still and berating herself was not using the important managerial skills she had access to from work. Braiker advised women to use their work techniques at home and on themselves, and to manage themselves better.[61] But even though these commentators stressed the powerful connections between women's public and private lives, they did not explore the disconnect between the collective action of the women's liberation movement and the solitary treatment of individual women for depression. Although depression was seen as due to disruptions in relationships, treatment focused on individuals and their intimate relationships, not on larger communities.

Though the message of treatment for depression cut against the primary methods of organization and activism as espoused by the feminist movement in the 1970s and 1980s, women did not seem to perceive this diagnosis as an expression of patriarchal physician authority.[62] Instead, women used the idea of depression as a way to call attention to their changing social circumstances and demand that their feelings be taken seriously. For example, some writers argued that physicians tended to dismiss childbirth blues as a transient clinical phenomenon because they did not really understand women's distress. Instead, women who discussed the experience among themselves came to the conclusion that postpartum depression was a real problem requiring real solutions.[63] In these interpretations of depression after childbirth, depression was not something to be uncovered by a physician, but rather was caused by the physician and the overtechnological medical system.[64] Indeed, because of the unique confluence of social problems for women, a number of writers—including women physicians—argued that depression was a disease of women and that treating depression was an important issue for women.[65]

The central role of relationships in many popular discussions of depression further distanced men. In popular accounts of families through the 1970s, men were hardly central to the emotional health of their families or other close relationships.[66] In the 1980s, men struggled to become engaged with their families in new ways and with different responsibilities.[67] Yet disruptions in intimate or family relationships did not seem to make men more vulnerable to depression since their presence within the family appeared to carry few emotional responsibilities. Indeed, many descriptions of depression in men were conveyed through the perspective of the afflicted men's wives or significant others. Most of the discussion about depression in men appeared in women's magazines, where the emphasis was on the ways that women needed to take care of and help to interpret their men. Boston-based researcher Myrna Weissman suggested in *Glamour* in 1980 that, if all else failed, a woman could give her man a copy of Percy Knauth's *A Season in Hell* to show him an example of another man who was depressed.[68] One psychologist contributor to the *Ladies' Home Journal* in 1984 suggested that men needed additional pampering during the holiday season because they were unable to cope with the conflicting emotions brought on by the season.[69] In many of these accounts of male depression written for a women's audience—presumably placed there on the theory that men would not go to the doctor unless women took them—men's depression became yet another disorder within women's intimate relationships.

But beyond instructions to understand men's feelings, women were often given somewhat conflicting messages about their male partner's emotional care. A psychologist educating readers in the *Ladies' Home Journal* in 1982 emphasized that wives should recognize depression in their husbands, and that the treatment involved more than trying to cheer them up. But at the same time that women were told to back off and give their husbands emotional space, they were also told that they had the responsibility to make sure their husbands sought the appropriate treatment.[70] A *McCall's* article in 1986 instructed women in what to do when their husbands were depressed—while the general thrust of the article was trying to educate women about when their husbands needed professional help, the article discussed a wide range of things that women needed to address in order to ensure their husband's mental health.[71]

Depression by the late 1980s was about relationships, not communities. While many perceived that America was in grave danger if the increasing rates of depression were not halted, the solution to depression lay in individuals (women) and their relationships with their intimate others. Instead of engaging in collective action to help their social circumstances, women were encouraged to work harder on their close relationships. Indeed, some writers even suggested that the women's movement had worsened conditions for women by causing an increase in depression and suicide.[72] But while women needed to work on themselves, depressed men needed to find women to interpret and help them. Even though the treatment of depression might have important political implications for women, social commentators emphasized the treatment of individual women. Women's social connectedness, as touted by advocates such as Maggie Scarf, appeared valuable to help women support each other in their depression, not for political purposes. The context of women's discontent that had been defined by Betty Friedan—women's isolation within a few intimate relationships—became the locus for treatment. Instead of the collective action urged by Friedan, American women by the 1970s and 1980s expressed their distress by increasingly getting help for depression.[73]

Consumption

While the ubiquity of modern pharmaceutical advertisements might suggest that consumption is an inevitable solution to depression, Americans have not always been eager to purchase in order to solve emotional problems. Indeed, in the first half of the twentieth century, a consumer ethos had not yet permeated popular discussions of mental health and nervousness, although large-scale manufacturing and national advertising were clearly growing influences in American culture. Instead, much public discussion indicated Americans' ongoing commitment to self-sacrifice and Puritan asceticism.[74] For many commentators, nervousness itself was evidence of the nation's problematic slide into decadence and overconsumption. Women were the worst offenders because it was their grasping for material possessions that led to nervousness in themselves and drove their husbands to be nervous because of the pressures of providing for their insatiable desires. Consumption was the cause, not the solution, for nervousness.

In the early twentieth century, many commentators deplored American women's efforts to look for solutions outside themselves: "Women who are suffering from 'Americanitis,' who are hurrying, worrying, grasping, struggling, tense or nerveless, distracted and unhappy, and uncomprehending. They are feeling about aimlessly for a new diversion, a new ambition, a new cult or a new doctor, not knowing that the kingdom of health, as well as the kingdom of heaven, is within them."[75] Most writers reported that American women became nervous because they put their energy into acquisition of new possessions or social standing. The rush of modernity—including the rush toward purchasing commodities—could be devastating to women because it changed their focus toward their communities and their families.

Early-twentieth-century commentators explicitly compared modern women's nervous strain with what they claimed was the lower stress for women of past generations.[76] As commentators complained, modern conditions put strain on women's natural roles, and writers fantasized about an ideal past in which men were hunters and women were gatherers.[77] One physician claimed that women's instincts to hoard would be frustrated if their modern men provided too much to them, and they would "miss inevitably and profoundly that wondrous fulfillment of woman's intended activity in upholding man in his daily labor of supply."[78] Commentators suggested that women's overconsumption led to modern ills such as an inability to balance occupation and leisure, care for self and others, and effectively run their households.[79] Further, women's overindulgence of their children could cause problems in the next generation, as writers argued that overindulgence produced neurotic children.[80]

Instead of purchasing products to prevent nervousness in the early decades of the century, commentators encouraged women to learn to manage themselves. As an added inducement, some writers argued that increased self-control would result in increased beauty—while unpleasant nervous traits, such as efforts to boss people around, were unattractive and needed to be countered in order to develop poise and grace.[81] Dr. Harvey W. Wiley, the founder of the Food and Drug Administration who also served as a medical adviser for *Good Housekeeping*, suggested to women that they needed to change their attitude about housekeeping in order to avoid nervousness. Instead of approaching housework as drudgery, Wiley advised women to approach each task with "artistic devotion."[82] Popular magazine writers consistently characterized nervous women as unattractive, querulous, and demanding, while women who were not nervous (or who had recovered) appeared poised and lovely. Annie Payson Call, a popular writer of a late-nineteenth-century handbook on appropriate regulation of body and rest, explained that nervousness indicated a system out of balance.[83] In an article in *Woman's Home Companion* in 1912, another woman commented that external appearance reflected not social class, but rather internal balance of energies. Nervous girls, regardless of their background, appeared awkward.[84] Although many of these instructions regarding emotional balance were similar to advertisements for beauty products that were in vogue during this time period, writers emphasized that women could enhance their beauty through emotional self-control.[85]

Consumption was also a problem for men in the early twentieth century because they felt compelled to work too hard to provide adequate luxuries for their families. One self-described neurasthetic man wrote in *American Magazine* that he had pushed himself because of his ideas about the work he had to accomplish as a man. As part of his recovery, he vowed that "never again will I listen to the promptings of the miserable fever of emulation that drives so many American men to sickness, despair, and madness."[86] What was clear to most commentators was that a man needed to work for his own good and for society, not overextend himself so that his family could have the latest modern conveniences.

But the role of consumption in emotional health changed significantly as depression appeared in popular magazines in the second half of the century. In the first decades of popular magazine discussions of low mood in women, writers encouraged a particular kind of consumption—shopping—to improve women's feelings about themselves. Early discussion around the blues in women's magazines suggested that women tended to engage in activities such as shopping in order to feel better.[87] Later writers also argued that women "naturally" helped themselves feel better by dressing better. In one study, a group of home economists surveyed women on the relationship between their mood and their dress. Contrary to their expectations, women who were depressed dressed better in order to feel better.[88]

As women's magazines increasingly provided self-help advice, writers regularly offered extensive lists of things that readers could do for themselves to help with their depression. A *Mademoiselle* article in 1974 contained seventy-nine things to do to "pick yourself up," while a 1977 *Redbook* article provided more instructions for what women should do to help when they were feeling depressed.[89] Most of the advice to depressed women included instructions to help them soothe themselves through positive experiences, including shopping (although women were cautioned not to overeat, since becoming overweight would further increase their depression).[90] Physician writers also promoted products to women to help their depression, including medications, structured therapy, and even electroshock therapy.[91] Writers' discussions of women's options about depression placed physicians' advice among other possible interventions, as women were encouraged to be active and intelligent consumers in the area of depression, as in so many other areas.[92]

Popular commentators who described depression around holidays— particularly the Christmas blues—emphasized that it was common for people to feel low around the rush and bustle of the holidays.[93] But while a cause for these low feelings appeared to be the rush to purchase, commentators did not advocate that people stop consuming in order to deal with the problem.[94] Instead, writers encouraged recognition of the problem and suggested ways for people to derive more meaning from the holiday.[95] The problem was not consumption; the problem was that the rampant consumption during the holidays did not seem to satisfy.[96] The treatment was to find ways to make the consumption more fulfilling.[97]

By the 1980s, women's magazines published many different formulas for treating a variety of low moods, from transient sadness to deep depression. These magazine accounts stressed both the need to seek out professional products (physician visits, medications, and structured therapy) as well as common things that women could do at home. During this time period, when magazine editors were attempting to capture and retain market share in an increasingly competitive field, the magazines themselves became part of the consumer solution. Magazines from *McCall's* to *Glamour* to *Vogue* offered women advice for eating, exercising, and shopping in order to deal with their bad feelings.[98] If nothing else, women who were feeling low could buy magazines that would give them advice on how to feel better.

The focus on individual women's experiences with depression further supported a consumerist model of depression: for a woman who needed help, the answer was in individual purchase of medications or psychotherapy.

The women's movement in the 1970s and 1980s had called for collective, social action to overcome inequality. Yet depression in medical and popular literatures of this time period made low mood in women, which writers admitted might have been indirectly caused by women's experiences with inequality, a personal problem in need of an individual solution. By the 1990s, with the rise of direct-to-consumer advertising for antidepressants, depression had clearly become another problem in search of a consumer solution. Indeed, products such as Prozac achieved their own celebrity, as the treatment for depression became as well known as the disease.[99]

The consumption model for depression was not nearly as comfortable a fit for men, however. One issue was that, in men's magazines as well as the psychiatrists' literature, men's low mood could be tied up with problems such as substance abuse or other physical abnormalities.[100] In addition, men with depression were rarely shown in their own accounts or those of others to have improved because of psychiatric treatments or because of self-help techniques—instead, men's accounts emphasized contingency in their recovery. Author Harlan Ellison reported that his case of depression appeared to be impervious to doctors' efforts to cure him.[101] Actor Robert Young, best known for his portrayal of the father in *Father Knows Best* (1950s) and as the title character in *Marcus Welby, M.D.* (1970s), acknowledged a thirty-year battle with depression that remitted only after long conversations with his wife.[102] Even writer William Styron, whose account of depression was probably the most widely publicized in the late 1980s and early 1990s, said that he recovered not because of drugs or psychotherapy but because of the atmosphere of the psychiatric hospital.[103] To the extent that men's depression appeared in popular magazines, it was not neat, tidy, or fixable with a consumer solution.[104]

Writer Louis Slovinsky's 1988 account of his depression illustrated some of the conflicts for men with depression in the popular literature. Slovinsky implied that real men did not get depressed, but also claimed that only men who had been depressed could understand depression in men. Further, he said that he relied on medications and thought that they helped him, but also blamed medications for causing him to be on the verge of suicide at one point in this treatment. The one clear element of Slovinsky's recovery was his engagement with Pennsylvania psychiatrist Aaron Beck's Cognitive Behavioral Therapy (CBT)—but Slovinsky's explanation of CBT emphasized how far removed it seemed from the usual professional advice: "Refreshingly free of shrink-speak, the treatment was short-term and useful." Slovinsky ended by pointing out that, in his depression, he joined a pantheon of other depressed men, including Dostoyevsky, Poe, Hawthorne, Darwin, Washington, Lincoln,

Churchill, Thomas Eagleton, and Edwin (Buzz) Aldrin Jr.[105] Slovinsky did not identify himself as a consumer but rather as a man in the company of other famous men (who happened to suffer from depression).[106]

Men's depression did not generate the same popular advice about consumption prompted by women's symptoms. But even on a philosophical level, men's writing about depression de-emphasized consumer culture in a way that harkened back to older descriptions of the problems of nervousness early in the century. Political commentator Harry Stein wrote a piece in *Esquire* in 1985 in which he proclaimed that those who came of age during John F. Kennedy's generation had lost heart with the struggle against huge, impersonal bureaucratic forces in the 1980s. He concluded that the culture was driven by empty values—that there was too much grasping for money. Instead, Stein advocated for self-control: "Genuine well-being is, in stark contrast, a matter of the heart and the guts; of a bedrock commitment to ideals; of striving, daily, on behalf of something larger than one's own comfort."[107] Stein suggested that men needed to make the choice to not be overwhelmed by the culture. Men's depression not only did not require consumption, but could in fact be seen as evidence of consumption run amok.

By the time new medications for depression were introduced in the late 1980s—most notoriously Prozac—depression appeared to be a widespread common disease that required consuming a product (or two or more) in order to treat it.[108] Popular magazine summaries of the illness, including one in *Reader's Digest* in 1990, emphasized that depression affected an enormous number of people. Certainly there were social factors: "These include the shifting roles of men and women, the flood of women into the workforce, and the acceleration of geographic movement that separates people from the support of their families and friends."[109] As a remedy for these social upheavals, authors recommended both professional advice and self-help techniques—many of which included some element of consumption. But perhaps most strikingly, at a time when commentators pointed out that Americans were suffering the emotional consequences of fewer family and community ties, magazines offered themselves as communities. By purchasing these magazines, reading about common problems, and taking the advice offered, more and more individuals—women as well as men—could try to buy their way to happiness.

Popular magazine images have been central to public understanding of depression as both an illness and as a way of conceptualizing the world. Their descriptions of depression have discussed what to do with the disease, but also have emphasized the gendered nature of relationships and happiness. While nervousness early in the century might have arisen out of the stresses of modern strivings, depression in the second half of the century became a disease of women's internal emotional life. Further, depression as a disease highlighted women's critical role of initiating and sustaining close relationships and ensuring the happiness of everyone around them. Women's obligations to sustain this happiness—like women's other obligations of keeping their homes clean and their children well educated—involved pursuit of commercial solutions to the problems of unhappiness. Is your man sad? Make sure he exercises and eats well. Are you down in the dumps? Get yourself to the mall and purchase something to make you feel better.

These popular discussions of depression illustrate the ways in which laypeople might have constructed their own meanings of depression out of physicians' descriptions of disease. But these magazine accounts also help to illustrate popular assumptions about gender, feelings, and relationships that were shared by the physicians who constructed the diagnosis of depression. Since physicians measured depression by patients' endorsement of feeling states, the difference in women's and men's mobilization of the language of feelings raises questions about how they might have responded to struc-tured interviews or symptom questionnaires. Indeed, popular representations of depression may have unintentionally deepened the differences between men and women in depression by highlighting the role of feelings. Magazine descriptions of women's easy emotional literacy provided a link between their introspection and solutions for depression. For men, however, magazine illustrations reinforced prevailing masculine disconnection from feeling states. Within American culture over the last several decades, what man would admit to feeling depressed?

The diagnosis of depression that emerged from medication trials in the 1960s and 1970s was based on criteria derived from psychiatrists' experiences with predominantly female patient populations. Many of these criteria required individuals to endorse specific feeling states in order to qualify for a diagnosis of depression. But though the authors of the diagnostic criteria intended for them to measure symptoms rather than social context, the language of feelings—especially as related to depression—has been limited largely to women. Popular magazine efforts to educate readers about depression further reinforced the idea that women are particularly vulnerable to depression, and also deepened the connection between the language of feelings and the diagnosis of depression.

Most of the changes in popular representations of mental illness that occurred during the emergence of depression as an illness both reflected and reinforced assumptions about women and how they would experience illness.

Those assumptions were so unquestioned that magazine writers happily and frequently repeated assurances that depression was something that particularly affected women (even when they sometimes discussed depression in men). In the last few years, there have been significant efforts to bring men's depression into public discussions, and the ways in which those narratives have jarred our popular understandings of the disease reveal how thoroughly depression has been shaped as a women's problem.

Real Men, Real Depression

In 2003, the National Institute of Mental Health (NIMH) launched a "Real Men. Real Depression." campaign to spread the word to men, who until now have not been a focus of depression research or education.[1] As the brochure that accompanied the campaign explained, men's depression can look different from women's: a man "may be grumpy or irritable, or have lost his sense of humor. He might drink too much or abuse drugs. It may be that he physically or verbally abuses his wife and his kids. He might work all the time, or compulsively seek thrills in high-risk behavior. Or, he may seem isolated, withdrawn, and no longer interested in the people or activities he used to enjoy."[2] The title of this campaign and the description of typical depressed men illustrate that the depression of the early twenty-first century—the diagnosis and the identity—does not fit men. The fact that depression is actively reshaped in the "Real Men. Real Depression." (note the emphasis with the punctuation in the campaign title) demonstrates the ways in which depression has been constructed as a women's disease.[3]

First, images of depression in men—in both the "Real Men" campaign and in recent magazine coverage of depressed men—stress that depression is a disease, not a feeling. Although education campaigns for depression have frequently emphasized the reality of disease, the campaign for educating men about depression focuses on biochemistry, with the implication that diagrams and pictures of molecules can better convey the disease to men. While a disease defined as a disorder of feelings might be real enough for women, the language of feelings has not been a part of men's repertoire in late-twentieth-century American culture. The "Real Men" brochure explains that modern "biomedical research" has demonstrated that depression is a real disease—and "brain imaging technologies are now allowing scientists to see how effective treatment with medication or psychotherapy is reflected in changes in brain activity." The reality of the disease can be seen, not just felt.[4] A 2007 *Newsweek* article on men and depression featured prominent pictures of brain images in positron emission tomography (PET) scans.[5] The "Real Men" campaign literature explicitly states that viewing depression as a "real" disease will help men get into treatment—they should be thinking about fighting depression with the same tools that are available to fight cancer.[6]

Not only does the "Real Men" campaign focus on brain pathology instead of emotional states, the campaign acknowledges that depressed men might have different symptoms from those listed in the fourth edition of the *Diagnostic and Statistical Manual* (*DSM-IV*). The "Real Men" campaign and the recent *Newsweek* presentations of depression include a list of eleven symptoms of depression relevant to men—but the *DSM-IV* only has nine criteria.[7] The extra two symptoms that are listed in the "Real Men" campaign are irritability (which had been in the *DSM-III* but was taken out) and unexplained physical symptoms. Indeed, the "Real Men" brochure explains that NIMH focus groups of men who helped to inform the campaign revealed that men were much more likely to talk about physical symptoms without realizing that they were describing depression.[8]

Finally, one of the most noticeable features of the "Real Men" campaign is that it includes abundant information from men who have been treated for depression. Instead of portraying men as consumers relying on expert advice, the campaign stresses men's opportunity to get answers from peers. These peers are indeed "real men"—they are listed by occupation and include a police officer, a diving champion, an air force sergeant, a lawyer, a publisher, and a writer. The stories, told by what reporters characterize as "macho men," reassure men that their masculinity will not be imperiled if they admit they are depressed.[9] Efforts to educate men about depression illustrate that the disease does not have to be an identity or label for men—but it does raise questions about the relationship among feelings, symptoms, emotions, and identity for both men and women.

The "Real Men. Real Depression." campaign attempts to reshape the diagnosis of depression to allow men to be included. But there are some problematic elements within this effort. The emphasis on men's ability to retain their identity as men while receiving depression treatment obscures an important part of these men's stories—as a *Time* article on this campaign revealed, all the men who ultimately received treatment for depression did so at the urging of their wives or girlfriends.[10] For men's depression as well as women's, women have the key role of consumer of professional goods and services. In addition, the "Real Men" campaign explains and to a certain extent excuses men's behavior—even aggression—with the argument that it is because of their depression. This clashes with our social and cultural expectations of men. As one man who was quoted in *Newsweek* explained, "I just thought I was a lousy husband and a miserable bastard and a drunk. . . . A mental illness? Me? I had no idea."[11] But does this reveal a problem with the diagnosis of depression or a problem with masculinity?[12]

Despite the NIMH's beautifully crafted effort to illustrate that depression is a disease that affects men, too, the recent popular literature on men's depression reinforces how much of a gendered phenomenon depression has become. Depression remains tied to consumption—and, in particular, women's consumption directed toward trying to resolve emptiness in their lives. The insistence with which the "Real Men" campaign emphasizes different aspects of depression does not eliminate the ways in which depression remains defined primarily as a disease of women. Women are told over and over again that if they feel bad, if they're having trouble sleeping or eating, or if they're not enjoying life, then it is a disease. In the 1960s, women objected to being told that their neuroses were due to their own failures. Now women are often eager to buy into the idea that the problem is within themselves, and many approach psychiatrists as suppliers of medications. Depression as a diagnosis allows women to externalize their problems—instead of struggling against the realities of strained marriages, inadequate compensation at work, and role stresses, they can take a pill. Women and physicians collude in seeing women's distress as something that can be managed with a prescription pad. Depression has become part of our mass market consumer society—it is a problem that can be solved with a product—and women are, in this area, as well as many others, active consumers.

Is there a problem with allowing women (and men if they want to) to act as consumers of mental health goods and services? The consumer focus with antidepressant medication in particular raises the question of whether an individual desire for improvement—based on dissatisfaction with life circumstances and given expression by a medication advertisement—should be enough for psychiatrists to prescribe medication.[13] Patient preference is certainly an important consideration for practitioners.[14] But is consumer demand the best way to make sure that people get treated for depression?

Depression has become commercialized—the process started with psychiatrists, was reinforced by enthusiasts, and has been exploited by pharmaceutical
companies.

As psychiatrist Peter Kramer first pointed out in 1993, several years after
the new medication Prozac helped to further popularize depression, the effect
of medications in American culture has been to alter how Americans view the
self. The language of brain chemistry, even more prevalent within American
popular culture after the introduction of a medication that named its neurochemical target (a selective serotonin reuptake inhibitor, or SSRI), seemed to
allow for the possibility that individuals could enhance themselves as they
treated their depression.[15] Kramer and other critics have argued, though, that
the idea of personality enhancement through medication creates a series of
challenging moral and ethical dilemmas.[16]

Further, our widespread medical and popular discussions about depression and its treatment have reinforced the idea that the individual is the
locus for intervention. Physicians continue to feel strongly that they need to
help individuals who express distress, despite awareness that patients' social
contexts might be contributing to their depression.[17] Yet the focus on the
individual misses patients' social context as a source of recovery and support.
Our diagnostic and disease model of depression emphasizes the individual
patient in relationship with a doctor (or health system)—not individuals in
their relationships to their communities. One recent major clinical trial of
antidepressants, the STAR*D trial, is a good example—the study does not
include the role of social networks for either stress or support, though the study
is intended to explore how patients respond to interventions of psychotherapy
or medications.[18] While psychoanalytic psychiatrists saw individuals in rich
tones and assessed their relationships, they still only identified the individual
patient as the locus for intervention. The biological and diagnostic psychiatrists
identified an individual patient as part of large statistical series who has some
statistical chance of response to any particular treatment.

Depression has important similarities to and differences from another
major group of diseases that achieved major significance in the latter part of the
twentieth century: eating disorders. Like depression, eating disorder categories
have been picking up momentum over the decades, and a greater number of
individuals than ever before can qualify for a diagnosis. Further, as historian
Joan Jacobs Brumberg points out, the symptom of food refusal has particular
meaning in a culture of food abundance.[19] In a similar way, depressive symptoms have a particular urgency in a society relentlessly set on happiness.
But though both depressive and eating disorders focus on the individual as

the source of the problem and of treatment, there is more ambivalence about treatment for eating disorders than for depression. While we as a society can easily tolerate—and even reward—likely (or confirmed) eating disorders in runway models and actresses, there is no longer a positive side for depression. Depression may be an understandable byproduct of life as a woman in today's society, but it comes with an injunction to treat.

There is a bitter irony about the fact that depression was solidified as a women's disease in the 1970s and 1980s. The first generation of feminists in the 1960s and 1970s had argued that women's unhappiness was a social problem that could be solved with collective action—consciousness-raising groups and political activism. Yet by the 1980s a woman's unhappiness was located solely within herself, and its treatment involved giving her medication or psychotherapy—and the diagnosis of depression was supported by feminists and researchers who argued that widespread recognition and treatment of depression was important to women. Although there remain real social, economic, cultural, and political issues for women, if they are unhappy with their situation the solution is to assume that it is disordered internal experience that can be corrected with a treatment for depression. While activists for men's equal treatment within mental health want men to receive attention for depression, it is not clear whether men are being offered help or further opportunities to focus on their internal lives rather than difficult work and social circumstances.

In 1975, Robert Woodruff, Paula Clayton, and Samuel Guze, prominent psychiatric researchers from Washington University, asked the question, "Is Everyone Depressed?" Woodruff and his colleagues noted that depression seemed to be everywhere, and they seriously assessed the possibility of widespread psychiatric disease by surveying relatives of depressed, hospitalized patients to see if the relatives were depressed. As it turned out, the relatives were *not* depressed, and so Woodruff and his group concluded that "if 'the mass of men lead lives of quiet desperation,' that despair is to be seen as philosophical, economic, or existential—not psychiatric in our sense. We believe the distinction is important and that failure to appreciate it has been a constant source of confusion for psychiatrists."[20] That Woodruff and his colleagues had to make a statement that *not all* human problems were necessarily due to psychiatric disorder illustrated how broad the claims for the diagnosis of depression had become in the heyday of depression research.

More than thirty years later, it is worthwhile asking again whether everyone is depressed. The depressive diagnoses criteria have expanded to include a huge range of feelings. Primary care physicians as well as psychiatrists are poised to diagnose and treat anyone who looks depressed. Pharmaceutical companies are aggressively promoting the view that any kind of emotional discomfort can be treated with a product—and they are happy to tell us the name of the products so we may ask our doctors about them. And now we have educational efforts directed at men that attempt to stretch the diagnosis even farther to accommodate men's experiences.

It remains to be seen whether the framers of *DSM-V* will consider changing criteria of major depressive disorder to include symptoms that the NIMH has said are critical to diagnosing men's depression, whether the pharmaceutical industry will expand its marketing efforts to include men, and whether researchers will continue to broaden the circumstances in which specific psychiatric interventions can be used for people. It also remains to be seen whether the enormous category of depression can continue to do all the medical and cultural work it is currently doing in explaining distress and providing a consumer solution. Unfortunately, there are few groups—outside of antipsychiatry activist groups—invested in shrinking the potential pool of people to be considered for the diagnosis of depression. Is everyone depressed? That question has not been completely answered, but the number of affected individuals appears to be growing by the minute.

Not only have physicians and consumers eagerly supported increasing diagnosis and treatment for depression in the United States, but a number of American researchers—and pharmaceutical industries—have emphasized the importance of global depression. But does depression look the same or play the same role in other societies?[21] European researchers have pointed out that even clinical trials of medications are affected by their national contexts, particularly around issues of patient selection. For example, European medication trials do not allow advertisements to and payments for patients who participate in trials (both of which are allowed in the United States). Further, the inducement of payment for treatment does not work in countries for which medical care is available to all.[22] The relatively small community of scholars exploring the major differences in expressions of distress across different cultures have illustrated the ways in which our symptom-based depression diagnostic criteria do not translate well into different settings.[23] Yet this cross-cultural research has not deterred American psychiatrists' and pharmaceutical industries' attempts to increase the global diagnosis of depression (based on *DSM* criteria) and increase the market for antidepressant medications.

As American society continues to emphasize community primarily within the confines of consumer culture, there is no mechanism to allow people to have a full range of feelings. Instead, in our mass market society, feelings have become things that need to be managed instead of experienced. There are enormous social problems in the United States—poverty, inadequate health insurance, racial injustice—and yet our focus on the individual has meant that we are treating unhappiness with medication instead of respecting it as a sign that we need to work together to solve social problems or shore up our community connections to help each other. The ubiquity of depression in our culture raises the question of whether women—or men if the NIMH campaign succeeds—are capable of living without having their lives propped up by chemistry.

Over the last century, numerous medical and popular writers have endeavored to find an answer for why Americans appeared to be vulnerable to certain mental disorders. Why, in a nation of abundance, opportunities for social mobility, and economic and religious freedoms, would there be large (and growing) rates of mental disease? While commentators have named different culprits over the decades—the decline of religion, the rise of consumerism, the disintegration of the family, among others—it may be that our attempts to fix emotional problems by focusing on individuals has exacerbated the problem.[24] Maybe it is our relentless individualism—in the pursuit of happiness, including the pursuit of psychiatric treatment—that fuels our particular American melancholy.

Notes

Introduction

1. American Psychiatric Association, *Diagnostic and Statistical Manual of Mental Disorders*, 4th ed., Text Revision ed. (Washington, D.C.: American Psychiatric Association, 2000), 356, 369–76.

2. Although some psychiatrists do practice psychotherapy, the typical practice today is for psychiatrists to be in charge of medications while other clinicians—usually social workers or psychologists—do therapy.

3. For an excellent account of the ways in which physicians and the pharmaceutical industry have redefined health and illness in diabetes, hypertension, and hypercholesterolemia, see Jeremy A. Greene, *Prescribing by Numbers: Drugs and the Definition of Disease* (Baltimore: Johns Hopkins University Press, 2007).

4. Recently, psychiatrists have become increasingly alarmed by what they have defined as treatment resistant depression—depression that persists despite months of treatment. This kind of depression, of course, has led to even more drug trials and calls for increased resources to deal with depression.

5. Greg Koski, "FDA and the Life-Sciences Industry: Business as Usual?" *Hastings Center Report* 34 (2004): 24–27.

6. The American Psychiatric Association was recently asked to reveal its specific financial relationships to pharmaceutical companies in the wake of increasing congressional concern about the possibility of bias. Benedict Carey and Gardiner Harris, "Psychiatric Group Faces Scrutiny Over Drug Industry Ties," *New York Times*, July 12, 2008.

7. Psychopharmacologist and historian David Healy has been an important and vocal critic of the role of the pharmaceutical industry in promoting medications for mental illness. See David Healy, *Let Them Eat Prozac: The Unhealthy Relationship between the Pharmaceutical Industry and Depression* (New York: New York University Press, 2004). See also Lawrence C. Rubin, "Merchandising Madness: Pills, Promises, and Better Living through Chemistry," *Journal of Popular Culture* 38 (2004): 369–83.

8. Ronald Bayer, *Homosexuality and American Psychiatry: The Politics of Diagnosis*, rev. ed. (Princeton, N.J.: Princeton University Press, 1987).

9. See especially Allan V. Horwitz, *Creating Mental Illness* (Chicago: University of Chicago Press, 2002). For a more recent exploration of depression in particular, see Allan V. Horwitz and Jerome C. Wakefield, *The Loss of Sadness: How Psychiatry Transformed Normal Sorrow into Depressive Disorder* (New York: Oxford University Press, 2007).

10. Market analysts estimated that 20 percent of the American population was being treated for depression at any one time, and they expected the rates to go up as the public was increasingly educated about depression. "Research & Markets: U.S. Antidepressant Market in Decline, Market Share of Generics to Increase, Report Says," *Health Insurance Week*, April 23, 2006, 103.

11. For critiques of *DSM*'s expansion into areas that are not real mental disease, see especially Jerome C. Wakefield, "Diagnosing DSM-IV—Part I: DSM-IV and the Concept of Disorder," *Behaviour Research and Therapy* 35 (1997): 633–49.

12. For the construction of illness in general, see, for example, Charles E. Rosenberg and Janet Golden, eds., *Framing Disease: Studies in Cultural History* (New Brunswick, N.J.: Rutgers University Press, 1992). For the construction of psychiatric illnesses, see Charles E. Rosenberg, "Contested Boundaries: Psychiatry, Disease, and Diagnosis," *Perspectives in Biology and Medicine* 49 (2006): 407–24; Allan Young, *The Harmony of Illusions: Inventing Post-Traumatic Stress Disorder* (Princeton, N.J.: Princeton University Press, 1995). There is considerable literature on the construction of older psychiatric ailments, particularly neurasthenia and hysteria. See, for example, Francis G. Gosling, *Before Freud: Neurasthenia and the American Medical Community, 1870–1910* (Urbana: University of Illinois Press, 1987); Mark S. Micale, *Approaching Hysteria: Disease and Its Interpretations* (Princeton, N.J.: Princeton University Press, 1995).

13. This is not to say, of course, that psychiatrists have completely eliminated psychoanalytic language or concepts from their thinking or practices. For an analysis of the ways in which psychoanalytic concepts affect medication treatments, see Jonathan Michel Metzl, *Prozac on the Couch: Prescribing Gender in the Era of Wonder Drugs* (Durham, N.C.: Duke University Press, 2003).

14. This accusation has been particularly leveled at psychiatrists around the diagnosis of Premenstrual Dysphoric Disorder (PMDD). See, for example, Paula J. Caplan, *They Say You're Crazy: How the World's Most Powerful Psychiatrists Decide Who's Normal* (Reading, Mass.: Addison-Wesley, 1995).

15. See Nancy Tomes, "Historical Perspectives on Women and Mental Illness," in *Women, Health, and Medicine in America*, ed. Rima D. Apple (New York: Garland, 1990), 143–72.

16. In order to locate medical articles, I did an issue-by-issue visual search of the entire century run of the *American Journal of Psychiatry*. I also looked at cited references from major articles on depression from the second half of the century and tracked them backward. For popular magazine articles, I relied on the *Reader's Guide to Periodical Literature*. (The search that formed the basis of the popular magazine sections of the book was completed prior to the full computer search capabilities of the *Reader's Guide*.) *Reader's Guide to Periodical Literature*, vol. 1900–1999 (New York: H. W. Wilson, 1900–1999).

17. Stanley W. Jackson, *Melancholia and Depression: From Hippocratic Times to Modern Times* (New Haven, Conn.: Yale University Press, 1986). See also Jennifer Radden, ed., *The Nature of Melancholy: From Aristotle to Kristeva* (New York: Oxford University Press, 2000); Andrew Solomon, *The Noonday Demon: An Atlas of Depression* (New York: Scribner, 2001).

18. Historian John Burnham has recently pointed out that a number of contingencies help to structure the medicalization of mental phenomenon. For an example of a condition that was not medicalized, see John C. Burnham, "The Syndrome of Accident Proneness (*Unfallneigung*): Why Psychiatrists Did Not Adopt and Medicalize It," *History of Psychiatry* 19 (2008): 251–74.

Chapter 1 — Prelude to Depression

1. See, for example, Hagop S. Akiskal, "Mood Disorders: Introduction and Overview," in *Kaplan & Sadock's Comprehensive Textbook of Psychiatry*, ed. Benjamin J. Sadock and Virginia A. Sadock (Philadelphia: Lippincott Williams & Wilkins, 2000), 1284–98. For a modern exploration of psychiatrists' past use of melancholia in a plea to bring back the concept, see Michael Alan Taylor and Max Fink, *Melancholia:*

The Diagnosis, Pathophysiology, and Treatment of Depressive Illness (New York: Cambridge University Press, 2006).

2. Judith Misbach and Henderikus Stam have argued that melancholia was medicalized in the late nineteenth and early twentieth centuries in America and Germany. See Judith Misbach and Henderikus J. Stam, "Medicalizing Melancholia: Exploring Profiles of Psychiatric Professionalization," *Journal of the History of the Behavioral Sciences* 42 (2006): 41–59.

3. See Andrew Abbott, *The System of Professions: An Essay on the Division of Expert Labor* (Chicago: University of Chicago Press, 1988), 280–314; Andrew Delano Abbott, "The Emergence of American Psychiatry, 1880–1930" (Ph.D. diss., University of Chicago, 1982). See also Edward M. Brown, "Neurology's Influence on American Psychiatry: 1865–1915," in *History of Psychiatry and Medical Psychology*, ed. Edwin R. Wallace IV and John Gach (New York: Springer, 2008), 519–31.

4. For the history of nineteenth- and twentieth-century American psychiatry, see especially the extraordinary body of work by Grob and a more recent overview by Shorter. Gerald N. Grob, *Mental Institutions in America: Social Policy to 1875* (New York: Free Press, 1973); Gerald N. Grob, *Mental Illness and American Society, 1875–1940* (Princeton, N.J.: Princeton University Press, 1983); Gerald N. Grob, *From Asylum to Community: Mental Health Policy in Modern America* (Princeton, N.J.: Princeton University Press, 1991); Edward Shorter, *A History of Psychiatry: From the Era of the Asylum to the Age of Prozac* (New York: John Wiley & Sons, 1997). For more on the nineteenth-century settings of psychiatry, see Nancy Tomes, *The Art of Asylum-Keeping: Thomas Story Kirkbride and the Origins of American Psychiatry* (Philadelphia: University of Pennsylvania Press, 1994); Ellen Dwyer, *Homes for the Mad: Life Inside Two Nineteenth-Century Asylums* (New Brunswick, N.J.: Rutgers University Press, 1987).

5. There is not yet a comprehensive history of American neurology. For some elements of this history, see Bonnie Ellen Blustein, "New York Neurologists and the Specialization of American Medicine," *Bulletin of the History of Medicine* 53 (1979): 170–83; Jeanne L. Brand, "Neurology and Psychiatry," in *The Education of American Physicians: Historical Essays*, ed. Ronald L. Numbers (Berkeley: University of California Press, 1980), 226–49.

6. Binghamton State Hospital was in New York. Cecil MacCoy, "Report of a Case of Melancholia Followed by Stupor Lasting Three Years and Eight Months; Recovery," *Journal of Nervous and Mental Disease* 28 (1901): 404–7. MacCoy's case was also discussed in Misbach and Stam, "Medicalizing Melancholia."

7. For more background on Jelliffe, see Paul Titus, ed., *Directory of Medical Specialists Certified by American Boards* (New York: Columbia University Press, 1940), 969; Derek Denny-Brown, Augustus S. Rose, and Adolph L. Satis, eds., *Centennial Anniversary Volume of the American Neurological Association, 1875–1975* (New York: Springer, 1975), 181–87.

8. Smith Ely Jelliffe and L. Pierce Clark, "The Work of a Neurological Dispensary Clinic," *Journal of Nervous and Mental Disease* 30 (1903): 482–88.

9. On Griesinger, see Shorter, *History of Psychiatry*, 72–81. On Kraepelin's influence in the United States, see Eugene Kahn, "The Emil Kraepelin Memorial Lecture," in *Epidemiology of Mental Disorder*, ed. Benjamin Pasamanick (Washington, D.C.: American Association for the Advancement of Science, 1959), 1–38.

10. Chas. W. Pilgrim, "The Study of a Year's Statistics," *American Journal of Insanity* 57 (1900): 47–55. For different local conditions in reference to Pilgrim, see Frederick

L. Hills, "A Statistical Study of One Thousand Patients," *American Journal of Insanity* 58 (1901): 151–65. William White, the superintendent of Government Hospital in Washington, D.C., argued that the extent of civilization, rather than the environment, per se, affected insanity and its distribution. See William A. White, "The Geographical Distribution of Insanity in the United States," *Journal of Nervous and Mental Disease* 30 (1903): 257–79.

11. See, for example, Edward Cowles, "Progress in the Clinical Study of Psychiatry," *American Journal of Insanity* 56 (1899): 109–22; Archibald Church and Frederick Peterson, "Manic-Depressive Insanity," in *Nervous and Mental Diseases* (Philadelphia: W. B. Saunders, 1919), 790–810. See also Emil Kraepelin, *Manic-Depressive Insanity and Paranoia*, ed. George M. Robertson, trans. R. Mary Barclay (Edinburgh: E. & S. Livingstone, 1921). Jackson pointed out, however, that the connection between these two mood states had been described long before Kraepelin. Jackson, *Melancholia and Depression*, 188–95.

12. See, for example, Charles G. Wagner, "The Treatment of Melancholia," *Medical Legal Journal* 19 (1901–2): 321–28; J. W. Wherry, "Melancholia: The Psychical Expression of Organic Fear," *American Journal of Insanity* 62 (1906): 369–406; George E. Price, "The Clinical Significance of Depression," *New York Medical Journal* 92 (1910): 313–15; Karl A. Menninger, "Melancholy and Melancholia," *Journal of the Kansas Medical Society* 21 (1921): 44–50.

13. For more on Beard's formulations, see George Miller Beard, *A Practical Treatise on Nervous Exhaustion (Neurasthenia), Its Symptoms, Nature, Sequences, Treatment* (New York: W. Wood, 1880); George Miller Beard, *American Nervousness, Its Causes and Consequences* (New York: G. P. Putnam's Sons, 1881). For historical discussion of Beard, see Charles E. Rosenberg, "George M. Beard and American Nervousness," in *No Other Gods: On Science and American Social Thought* (Baltimore: Johns Hopkins University Press, 1976), 98–108; Gosling, *Before Freud*; Marijke Gijswijt-Hofstra and Roy Porter, eds., *Cultures of Neurasthenia from Beard to the First World War* (Amsterdam: Rodopi, 2001).

14. See Tom Lutz, "Neurasthenia and Fatigue Syndromes: Social Section," in *A History of Clinical Psychiatry: The Origin and History of Psychiatric Disorders*, ed. German E. Berrios and Roy Porter (New York: New York University Press, 1995), 533–44.

15. See, for example, H. E. Allison, "Simple Melancholia and Its Treatment," *Medical Record* 51 (1897): 39–41. "Simple depression" did appear in neurologists' (but not psychiatrists') official nomenclature and disease classification in the 1930s. H. B. Logie, ed., *A Standard Classified Nomenclature of Disease* (New York: Commonwealth Fund, 1933).

16. "Allopathic" was the descriptor given to regular physicians in the nineteenth century in the context of their competition with other practitioners, including homeopaths. Paul Starr, *The Social Transformation of American Medicine* (New York: Basic Books, 1982), 100. Allopathic treatment was the treatment by opposite, while homeopathic remedies involved administering microdoses of the same agent that presumably caused the symptoms. For more on allopathic medicine, see William G. Rothstein, *American Medical Schools and the Practice of Medicine* (New York: Oxford University Press, 1987). For more on the history of alternatives to allopathic medicine, see James C. Whorton, *Nature Cures: The History of Alternative Medicine in America* (New York: Oxford University Press, 2002).

17. See, for example, George Stockton, "Melancholia and Its Treatment," *Philadelphia Medical Journal* 8 (1901): 571–73; Shepherd Ivory Franz and G. V. Hamilton, "The

Effects of Exercise Upon the Retardation in Conditions of Depression," *American Journal of Insanity* 62 (1905): 239–56. On the potential dangers of these treatments, see, for example, Adolf Meyer, "On Some Terminal Diseases in Melancholia," *American Journal of Insanity* 59 (1902): 83–89. For some of the dangers in somatic therapies in the hospital setting in the first half of the century, see Andrew Scull, *Madhouse: A Tragic Tale of Megalomania and Modern Medicine* (New Haven, Conn.: Yale University Press, 2005).

18. See, for example, L. Pierce Clark, "Some Therapeutic Considerations of Periodic Mental Depressions," *Medical Record* 93 (1918): 223–29. Of course, the nineteenth-century treatment for neurasthenia, the rest cure, had become well known in American literary circles after Charlotte Perkins Gilman's experiences with Phila-delphia neurologist S. Weir Mitchell, who pioneered this treatment. See Charlotte Perkins Gilman, *The Yellow Wallpaper* (Boston: Small & Maynard, 1899); Barbara Sicherman, "The Uses of a Diagnosis: Doctors, Patients, and Neurasthenia," *Journal of the History of Medicine and Allied Sciences* 32 (1977): 33–54; David G. Schuster, "Personalizing Illness and Modernity: S. Weir Mitchell, Literary Women, and Neur-asthenia, 1870–1914," *Bulletin of the History of Medicine* 79 (2005): 695–722.

19. See, for example, Warren L. Babcock, "On the Treatment of Acute and Curable Forms of Melancholia," *International Medical Magazine* 9 (1900): 1–6.

20. See, for example, Ross McC. Chapman, "The Control of Sleeplessness," *American Journal of Psychiatry* 80 (1924): 491–502.

21. See, for example, Sidney I. Schwab, "The Use of Social Intercourse as a Therapeutic Agent in the Psychoneuroses, a Contribution to the Art of Psychotherapy," *Journal of Nervous and Mental Disease* 34 (1907): 497–503; L. Pierce Clark, "The Psycho-logic Treatment of Retarded Depressions," *American Journal of Insanity* 75 (1919): 407–10.

22. Meyer Solomon, "A Neglected but Important Cause of Mental Depression," *Chicago Medical Record* 37 (1915): 635–39, quote from 639. See also Charles F. Read, "Mental Depression," *Illinois Medical Journal* 33 (1918): 253–57. For informa-tion about Solomon, see *American Medical Directory*, 6th ed. (Chicago: American Medical Association, 1918), 472; Titus, *Directory of Medical Specialists*, 940.

23. Clarence B. Farrar, "On the Methods of Later Psychiatry," *American Journal of Insanity* 61 (1905): 437–66, quote from 439. See also William A. White, "Types in Mental Disease," *Journal of Nervous and Mental Disease* 33 (1906): 254–64.

24. See, for example, P. M. Wise, "Presidential Address, Delivered at the Annual Meeting of the American Medico-Psychological Association, Held at Milwaukee, Wis., June 11–14, 1901," *American Journal of Insanity* 58 (1901): 79–95. Some argued that mental symptoms were manifestations of a single (or a few) disease process(es), on the model of general paresis. See H. A. Tomlinson, "The Unity of Insanity," *American Journal of Insanity* 63 (1906): 155–66; E. Stanley Abbot, "Forms of Insanity in Five Years' Admissions to, and Discharges from, the Hospitals for the Insane in Massachusetts," *American Journal of Insanity* 66 (1909): 111–22. On the role of physiology and disease, see Gerald L. Geison, ed., *Physiology in the American Context, 1850–1940* (Baltimore: American Physiological Society, 1987). On the increasing application of the germ theory to broader areas of medicine and society, see Nancy Tomes, *The Gospel of Germs: Men, Women, and the Microbe in American Life* (Cambridge, Mass.: Harvard University Press, 1998).

25. Lewellys F. Barker, "The Relations of Internal Medicine to Psychiatry," *American Journal of Psychiatry* 71 (1914): 13–28.

26. For a discussion of classification in the context of other professional concerns, see, for example, George L. Walton, "The Classification of Psycho-Neurotics, and the Obsessional Element in Their Symptoms," *Journal of Nervous and Mental Disease* 34 (1907): 489–96.

27. See, for example, August Hoch, "On the Clinical Study of Psychiatry," *American Journal of Insanity* 57 (1900): 281–95; E. Stanley Abbot, "The Criteria of Insanity and the Problems of Psychiatry," *American Journal of Insanity* 59 (1902): 1–16.

28. See, for example, Henry M. Hurd, "Psychiatry as a Part of Preventive Medicine," *American Journal of Insanity* 65 (1908): 17–24; William L. Russell, "The Widening Field of Practical Psychiatry," *American Journal of Insanity* 70 (1913): 459–66. Historian Elizabeth Lunbeck has analyzed the beginnings of psychiatrists' efforts to expand their professional authority beyond the hospital. Elizabeth Lunbeck, *The Psychiatric Persuasion: Knowledge, Gender, and Power in Modern America* (Princeton, N.J.: Princeton University Press, 1994).

29. The career of Albert Moore Barrett provides a good example of the fluid boundaries between laboratory science, neurology, and psychiatry. Barrett was trained as a neurologist and as a pathologist (he published on autopsy findings), but also chaired a psychiatry department, was president of the American Psychiatric Association in 1921, and was president of the American Neurological Association in 1936. See Albert Moore Barrett Papers, Bentley Historical Library, University of Michigan, Ann Arbor; Albert M. Barrett, "A Case of Pure Word-Deafness with Autopsy," *Journal of Nervous and Mental Disease* 37 (1910): 73–92; Albert M. Barrett, "A Case of Alzheimer's Disease with Unusual Neurological Disturbances," *Journal of Nervous and Mental Disease* 40 (1913): 361–74.

30. For the formation of the American Board, see Walter Freeman, Franklin Ebaugh, and David A. Boyd, "The Founding of the American Board of Psychiatry and Neurology, Inc.," *American Journal of Psychiatry* 115 (1959): 769–78. For the transition within neurology, see Russell N. DeJong, *A History of American Neurology* (New York: Raven Press, 1982). As Tom Lutz has pointed out, neurasthenia as an illness had mostly disappeared within American medicine by this time period. Tom Lutz, "Varieties of Medical Experience: Doctors and Patients, Psyche and Soma in America," in Gijswijt-Hofstra and Porter, *Cultures of Neurasthenia*, 51–76.

31. See, for example, J. C. Whitehorn and Gregory Zilboorg, "Present Trends in American Psychiatric Research," *American Journal of Psychiatry* 90 (1933): 303–12; Willard C. Rappleye, "Comments on Psychiatry," *American Journal of Psychiatry* 91 (1934): 241–46.

32. Sigmund Freud, "Mourning and Melancholia," in *The Standard Edition of the Complete Psychological Works of Sigmund Freud* (London: Hogarth Press, 1917), 237–58.

33. See, for example, Sandor Rado, "The Problem of Melancholia," *International Journal of Psychoanalysis* 9 (1928): 420–38; Gregory Zilboorg, "Depressive Reactions Related to Parenthood," *American Journal of Psychiatry* 87 (1931): 927–62; J. Harnik, "Introjection and Projection in the Mechanism of Depression," *International Journal of Psychoanalysis* 13 (1932): 425–32; Paul Federn, "The Reality of the Death Instinct, Especially in Melancholia," *Psychoanalytic Review* 19 (1932): 129–51; Joseph R. Blalock, "Mental Mechanisms in Depression," *Psychiatric Quarterly* 8 (1934): 98–110; Kiyoyasu Marui, "The Process of Introjection in Melancholia," *Journal of Psychoanalysis* 16 (1935): 49–58; Georg Gero, "The Construction of Depression," *International Journal of Psychoanalysis* 17 (1936): 423–61; Chester L.

Carlisle, "Depressions Which Followed Apparent Success," *American Journal of Psychiatry* 95 (1938): 729–32.

34. Paul Schilder, "Clinical Studies on Particular Types of Depressive Psychoses—Their Differential Diagnosis from Schizophrenic Pictures and Some Remarks on the Psychology of Depressions," *Journal of Nervous and Mental Disease* 80 (1934): 501–27, 658–83.

35. As Boston psychiatrist Abraham Myerson explained in 1939 with his survey of American psychiatrists and neurologists, members of both groups were somewhat interested in, but not necessarily in complete agreement with, the concepts and approaches of Freudian psychoanalysis. Abraham Myerson, "The Attitude of Neurologists, Psychiatrists and Psychologists towards Psychoanalysis," *American Journal of Psychiatry* 96 (1939): 623–41. For more history of the combination of somatic treatments and psychoanalytic perspectives, see Jonathan H. Sadowsky, "Beyond the Metaphor of the Pendulum: Electroconvulsive Therapy, Psychoanalysis, and the Styles of American Psychiatry," *Journal of the History of Medicine and Allied Sciences* 61 (2006): 1–25.

36. Several authors extolled the benefits of hematoporphyrin, a by-product of blood discovered by a German physician, which seemed to energize animals. J. Huehnerfeld, "The Hematoporphyrin Treatment of Melancholia and Endogenous Depression," *American Journal of Psychiatry* 92 (1936): 1323–30. Historian Nicholas Rasmussen has recently pointed out that amphetamines were used as antidepressants in this time period, but primarily in outpatient practice. Nicolas Rasmussen, "Making the First Anti-Depressant: Amphetamine in American Medicine, 1929–1950," *Journal of the History of Medicine and Allied Sciences* 61 (2006): 288–323. I did not find mention of amphetamines in my research, but the idea of stimulating sluggish patients was certainly described in the medical literature I analyzed. See also Nicholas Rasmussen, *On Speed: The Many Lives of Amphetamine* (New York: New York University Press, 2008).

37. For shock therapies, see, for example, William C. Menninger, "An Evaluation of Metrazol Treatment," *Bulletin of the Menninger Clinic* 4 (1940): 95–104; Lothar B. Kalinowsky and Harry J. Worthing, "Results with Electric Convulsive Therapy in 200 Cases of Schizophrenia," *Psychiatric Quarterly* 17 (1943): 144–53; Harry J. Worthing, Newton Bigelow, Richard Binzley, and Henry Brill, "The Organization and Administration of a State Hospital Insulin-Metrazol-Electric Shock Therapy Unit," *American Journal of Psychiatry* 99 (1943): 692–97. For an exemplary discussion of somatic treatments in the first half of the century, see Joel Braslow, *Mental Ills and Bodily Cures: Psychiatric Treatment in the First Half of the Twentieth Century* (Berkeley: University of California Press, 1997). On the history of insulin treatment, see Deborah Blythe Doroshow, "Performing a Cure for Schizophrenia: Insulin Coma Therapy on the Wards," *Journal of the History of Medicine and Applied Sciences* 62 (2007): 213–43. On the history of electroconvulsive therapy, see Edward Shorter and David Healy, *Shock Therapy: A History of Electroconvulsive Treatment in Mental Illness* (New Brunswick, N.J.: Rutgers University Press, 2007).

38. Jack Pressman provided a compelling account that explained why psychiatrists of the time thought this treatment was effective. Jack D. Pressman, *Last Resort: Psychosurgery and the Limits of Medicine* (New York: Cambridge University Press, 1998). For some more critical accounts of lobotomy, see Jack El-Hai, *The Lobotomist: A Maverick Medical Genius and His Tragic Quest to Rid the World of Mental Illness* (Hoboken, N.J.: John Wiley & Sons, 2005); Elliot S. Valenstein, *Great and Desperate*

Cures: The Rise and Decline of Psychosurgery and Other Radical Treatments for Mental Illness (New York: Basic Books, 1986).

39. Psychiatrists worked with their professional organization (the American Medico-Psychological Association, shortly to be renamed the American Psychiatric Association) and the National Committee for Mental Hygiene (NCMH) to outline and distribute a classification system for mental institutions in 1918, a system that was put into use in the 1922 census (though it was not widely used in clinical practice). Committee on Statistics of the American Medico-Psychological Association and Bureau of Statistics of the National Committee for Mental Hygiene, *Statistical Manual for the Use of Institutions for the Insane* (New York: National Committee for Mental Hygiene, 1918). The American Neurological Association (ANA) produced a disease classification system in 1928 that attempted to classify all of the diseases that could affect the nervous system or mental states. American Neurological Association, *A Classification of Neurological, Psychiatric and Endocrine Disorders* (New York: American Neurological Association, 1928).

40. For some of the history of statistics, see Theodore M. Porter, *The Rise of Statistical Thinking, 1820–1900* (Princeton, N.J.: Princeton University Press, 1986); Harry M. Marks, "Trust and Mistrust in the Marketplace: Statistics and Clinical Research, 1945–1960," *History of Science* 38 (2000): 343–55.

41. Haven Emerson and George Baehr, "Preface," in Logie, *Standard Classified Nomenclature of Disease*, xi–xvii. The medical organizations originally invited to the conference at the New York Academy of Medicine included the American College of Surgeons, the American Heart Association, the American Hospital Association, the American Statistical Association, the American Surgical Association, the Association of American Physicians, the Bureau of the Census, and the medical departments of the army and navy. The insurance companies that assisted in funding the project were the Metropolitan Life Insurance Company, the Prudential Insurance Company of America, and the Connecticut General Life Insurance Company. For biographical information on Emerson, see D. O. Powell, "Haven Emerson," *Dictionary of American Medical Biography*, vol. 1, ed. Martin Kaufman, Stuart Galishoff, and Todd L. Savitt (Westport, Conn.: Greenwood Press, 1983), 231.

42. Leslie B. Hohman, "A Review of One Hundred and Forty-four Cases of Affective Disorders—After Seven Years," *American Journal of Psychiatry* 94 (1937): 303–8, quote from 303. Although he identified himself as a psychiatrist, Hohman was a member of both the APA and the ANA. *American Medical Directory*, 13th ed. (Chicago: Press of the American Medical Association, 1934), 733.

43. Although anxiety was also a topic in psychiatric literature, articles about depression began to significantly outnumber articles about anxiety in the *American Journal of Psychiatry* by the 1960s and 1970s. Further, anxiety disorders in *DSM-III* were also referred to as neuroses. American Psychiatric Association, *Diagnostic and Statistical Manual of Mental Disorders*, 3rd ed. (Washington, D.C.: American Psychiatric Association, 1980), 225–39.

44. For general histories of popular culture and models of interaction among professional and popular literatures, see John Fiske, *Understanding Popular Culture* (New York: Routledge, 1989); Richard Wightman Fox and T. J. Jackson Lears, eds., *The Power of Culture: Critical Essays in American History* (Chicago: University of Chicago Press, 1993).

45. One newspaper editor who spoke before the American Medico-Psychological

Association in 1915 explained that public opinion, particularly the phenomenon of the mob mind, was analogous to mental illness and asked psychiatrists to help manage it. Douglas Southall Freeman, "Publicity and the Public Mind," *American Journal of Insanity* 72 (1915): 17–33.

46. Practitioners who publicized their efforts ran the risk of being labeled as quacks during this time period. See James Harvey Young, *The Medical Messiahs: A Social History of Health Quackery in Twentieth-Century America* (Princeton, N.J.: Princeton University Press, 1967).

47. For the classic reference on American popular periodicals, see Frank Luther Mott, *A History of American Magazines*, 5 vols. (Cambridge, Mass.: Harvard University Press, 1938–68).

48. As Jackson Lears has argued, this time period was "the beginning of a shift from a Protestant ethos of salvation through self-denial toward a therapeutic ethos stressing self-realization in this world—an ethos characterized by an almost obsessive concern with psychic and physical health defined in sweeping terms." T. J. Jackson Lears, "From Salvation to Self-Realization: Advertising and the Therapeutic Roots of the Consumer Culture, 1880–1930," in *The Culture of Consumption: Critical Essays in American History, 1880–1980*, ed. Richard Wightman Fox and T. J. Jackson Lears (New York: Pantheon Books, 1983), 3–38, quote from 4.

49. See, for example, Graeme M. Hammond, "Nerves and the American Woman," *Harper's Bazar* [sic], July 1906, 590–93. For a general audience description of nervous phenomena and their treatments, see Paul Dubois, *The Psychic Treatment of Nervous Disorders (The Psychoneuroses and Their Moral Treatment)*, trans. Smith Ely Jelliffe and William A. White, 4th ed. (New York: Funk & Wagnalls, 1908).

50. See, for example, Charles Phelps Cushing, "The Business Man with 'Nerves,'" *World's Work*, September 1916, 569–74.

51. For physician-authored accounts that provided opportunities for readers to identify as potential patients, see Leonard Keene Hirshberg, "The Tyranny of Fear," *Harper's Weekly*, November 16, 1912, 20; Burton J. Hendrick, "The Disease of Fear and Its Cure," *McClure's*, July 1914, 137–48.

52. Henry Smith Williams, "Are Your Nerves in Tune?" *Good Housekeeping*, February 1914, 186–93, quote from 187.

53. See, for example, William S. Sadler, *Worry and Nervousness, or the Science of Self-Mastery* (Chicago: A. C. McClurg, 1915).

54. See, for example, "The Diagnosis of Neurasthenia," *Current Literature*, October 1900, 433–44; "The Sole Test of Sanity," *Literary Digest*, November 16, 1918, 25.

55. W. F. Becker, "Morbid Sense of Injury," *Popular Science*, March 1900, 596–602, quote from 602.

56. Carl W. Sawyer, "Give Your Brain a Chance," *Rotarian*, January 1936, 27–30, quote from 27.

57. Henrik G. Peterson, "Unrecognized Insanity: A Public and Individual Danger," *Arena*, November 1906, 508–15.

58. J. M. Buckley, "How to Safeguard One's Sanity," *Century*, July 1900, 375–80.

59. See, for example, "Passing of 'Insanity,'" *Literary Digest*, March 21, 1914, 616–17.

60. Psychiatrists had also received popular attention for their work with shell shock victims and recruit screening during World War I. See, for example, "Music for Shattered Minds," *Literary Digest*, June 10, 1916, 1742; Pearce Bailey, "Psychiatry and the Army," *Harper's Magazine*, July 1917, 251–57; Pearce Bailey, "Prevention of Nervous Casualties," *New Republic*, January 5, 1918, 275–76. For the post–World

War II rise of American enthusiasm for psychiatry and psychology, see Ellen Herman, *The Romance of American Psychology: Political Culture in the Age of Experts* (Berkeley: University of California Press, 1995).

61. "In Uniform and Their Right Minds," *Time*, June 1, 1942, 36–38.

62. See, for example, "Spit It Out, Soldier," *Time*, September 13, 1943, 60–62; Don Wharton, "Twilight Healing for Shell-Shocked Veterans," *Reader's Digest*, July 1945, 89–92; M. J. Farrell, "Plain Truths About the 'N.P.s,'" *Rotarian*, October 1944, 55–57; Frederick C. Painton, "There Is No Such Thing as Shell Shock," *Reader's Digest*, October 1943, 59–63.

63. Frank N. Trager, "Some Don't Wear the Purple Heart," *Nation*, October 6, 1945, 335–37; "Guadalcanal Neurosis," *Time*, May 24, 1943, 39–42; "Isle of Nightmare," *Newsweek*, May 24, 1943, 88–89; "War Nerves," *Newsweek*, January 4, 1943, 65.

64. S. W. Morris, "Sports Heal War Neuroses," *Recreation*, October 1945, 39.

65. "Air Raids Test Marriage," *Time*, August 18, 1941, 56; "Heartsickness," *Time*, January 29, 1945, 65; J. C. Furnas, "Meet Ed Savickas," *Ladies' Home Journal*, February 1945, 141–44; Leslie B. Hohman, "Combat Fatigue," *Ladies' Home Journal*, February 1945, 146–47.

66. See, for example, "The Heavy-Laden," *Time*, February 7, 1944, 44, 47–48. For more on the history of narcosynthesis and psychoanalytic psychiatric practice during the war, see Nathan G. Hale Jr., *The Rise and Crisis of Psychoanalysis in the United States: Freud and the Americans, 1917–1985* (New York: Oxford University Press, 1995), 191–98. The experimental animal basis of this kind of treatment was also provided to readers of popular magazines. See "Catatonic Cats," *Time*, June 8, 1942, 54–55; "Dog's Neurosis," *Newsweek*, August 21, 1944, 80–82.

67. For more information about American psychiatry and World War II, see Gerald N. Grob, "World War II and American Psychiatry," *Psychohistory Review* 19 (1990): 41–69; Paul Wanke, "American Military Psychiatry and Its Role among Ground Forces in World War II," *Journal of Military History* 63 (1999): 127–46.

68. Maurice Zolotow, "Doctors of Dilemmas," *Collier's*, September 9, 1944, 73, 78–79, quote from 78. On the dangerous combination of war and already weak intellectual or emotional processes, see "War and the Mind," *Time*, January 4, 1943, 44.

69. See, for example, S. T. Rorer, "What Nervous People Should Eat," *Ladies' Home Journal*, February 1909, 40; Abraham Myerson, "The Riddle of Abnormal Minds. VI. A Program of Mental Hygiene," *Independent*, December 25, 1926, 737–39; "Chewers and Chewing," *Independent*, October 31, 1907, 1072–73; "Sports as Remedies for Neurasthenia," *Review of Reviews*, October 1912, 501–2.

70. John K. Mitchell, "Self Help for Nervous Women," *Harper's Bazar*, August 1901, 382–85, quote from 383.

71. Louise Collier Willcox, "Crises de Nerfs," *Harper's Weekly*, June 21, 1913, 5; "The Nerve Doctor," *Living Age*, August 30, 1913, 561–63; Maxine Davis, "You've Got Your Nerves!" *Pictorial Review*, June 1938, 18–19, 64–65.

72. See Samuel McComb, "Nervousness in Women: Its Cause and Cure," *Harper's Bazar*, October 1907, 962–64; "Mental Medicine," *Independent*, June 25, 1908, 1460–61; Samuel McComb, "My Experience with Nervous Sufferers," *Harper's Bazar*, January 1910, 29. In general, McComb's authority seemed to be fairly well accepted by other popular writers on the subject (including physicians), although one neurologist in 1910 complained about what he perceived to be McComb's claim that the Emmanuel Movement was the only one that appropriately treated nervous disorders. See Ralph Wallace Reed, "The Emmanuel Movement," *Everybody's*

Magazine, May 1910, 713–14. For more on the Emmanuel Movement's advice to patients, see Elwood Worcester, Samuel McComb, and Isador H. Coriat, *Religion and Medicine: The Moral Control of Nervous Disorders* (New York: Moffat, Yard, 1908); Elwood Worcester and Samuel McComb, *Body, Mind and Spirit* (New York: Charles Scribner's Sons, 1932).

73. See, for example, George Lincoln Walton, "Those Nerves: Character-Leakage," *Lippincott's Magazine*, September 1909, 363–65; George Lincoln Walton, "Those Nerves: Sidetractibility," *Lippincott's Magazine*, August 1909, 202–4.

74. See, for example, Annie Payson Call, "What Is It That Makes Me So Nervous?" *Ladies' Home Journal*, June 1911, 14; H. Addington Bruce, "Selfishness and Your Nerves," *Good Housekeeping*, October 1916, 39–40, 116–18; Friedrich Jensen, "Who Is Neurotic?" *Atlantic Monthly*, December 1935, 692–94; Anne Bryan McCall, "The Girl Who Is Nervous," *Woman's Home Companion*, June 1912, 27; "Death in Incurable Disease," *Independent*, December 12, 1912, 1385–87.

75. Samuel McComb, "Nervous Poise and How to Get It," *Harper's Bazar*, October 1909, 1003–5. See also William S. Sadler, "Ways to Work Out Your Own Mind Cure," *American Magazine*, August 1924, 41, 126–31.

76. Clifford Beers, *A Mind That Found Itself* (New York: Doubleday, 1908). While Beers was originally interested in correcting problems in mental hospitals, his energy and enthusiasm were harnessed by Johns Hopkins psychiatry chairman Adolf Meyer to address the general issue of insanity prevention. Norman Dain, *Clifford W. Beers, Advocate for the Insane* (Pittsburgh: University of Pittsburgh Press, 1980). For histories of the mental hygiene movement, particularly its relationship to work with children, see Theresa R. Richardson, *The Century of the Child: The Mental Hygiene Movement and Social Policy in the United States and Canada* (Albany: State University of New York Press, 1989); Margo Horn, *Before It's Too Late: The Child Guidance Movement in the United States, 1922–1945* (Philadelphia: Temple University Press, 1989).

77. Howard J. Faulkner and Virginia D. Pruitt, eds., *Dear Dr. Menninger: Women's Voices from the Thirties* (Columbia: University of Missouri Press, 1997). For background on Menninger and his public reputation, see Lawrence J. Friedman, *Menninger: The Family and the Clinic* (New York: Knopf, 1990).

78. For a fascinating study of the history of bad habits, see John C. Burnham, *Bad Habits: Drinking, Smoking, Taking Drugs, Gambling, Sexual Misbehavior, and Swearing in American History* (New York: New York University Press, 1993).

79. George K. Pratt, "Education and Interpretation: Two Essentials in a Mental Hygiene Program," *American Journal of Psychiatry* 80 (1924): 463–74. Psychiatrists were certainly not the first mental health professionals to become involved in mass marketing. John Watson, the founder of behaviorism, went to work for an advertising firm in the 1920s, and eventually became the vice president. He saw advertising as a natural outgrowth of his work in applied psychology. Kerry W. Buckley, "The Selling of a Psychologist: John Broadus Watson and the Application of Behavioral Techniques to Advertising," *Journal of the History of the Behavioral Sciences* 18 (1982): 207–21.

80. Herman, *Romance of American Psychology*. See also Hale, *Rise and Crisis of Psychoanalysis*, 276–99.

81. See Howard Markel, *Quarantine! East European Jewish Immigrants and the New York City Epidemics of 1892* (Baltimore: Johns Hopkins University Press, 1997). On health fears of immigrants, see Alan M. Kraut, *Silent Travelers: Germs, Genes, and*

the Immigrant Menace (Baltimore: Johns Hopkins University Press, 1995). For an exploration of immigrants in popular culture, see Rachel Rubin and Jeffrey Melnick, *Immigration and American Popular Culture: An Introduction* (New York: New York University Press, 2006).

82. The historical literature on eugenics is considerable. See, for example, Ian Robert Dowbiggin, *Keeping America Sane: Psychiatry and Eugenics in the United States and Canada, 1880–1940* (Ithaca, N.Y.: Cornell University Press, 1997); Daniel J. Kevles, *In the Name of Eugenics: Genetics and the Uses of Human Heredity* (Berkeley: University of California Press, 1985); Martin S. Pernick, *The Black Stork: Eugenics and the Death of "Defective" Babies in American Medicine and Motion Pictures since 1915* (New York: Oxford University Press, 1996); Alexandra Minna Stern, *Eugenic Nation: Faults and Frontiers of Better Breeding in Modern America* (Berkeley: University of California Press, 2005).

83. For a powerful analysis of the late-nineteenth and early-twentieth-century confrontations with modern life and its meanings, see T. J. Jackson Lears, *No Place of Grace: Antimodernism and the Transformation of American Culture, 1880–1920* (Chicago: University of Chicago Press, 1981).

84. Jean Williams, "Help for the Nervous Woman," *Woman's Home Companion*, November 1910, 49.

85. See, for example, Samuel McComb, "Some Causes of Nervousness," *Harper's Bazar*, July 1909, 646–49; Agnes Repplier, "The Nervous Strain," *Atlantic Monthly*, August 1910, 198–201; "Nerve Diseases Caused by Success in Life," *Current Opinion*, December 1918, 380. A professor Munsterberg argued, however, that modern conveniences would lessen nervous strain. See "The Age of Nerves," *Living Age*, November 19, 1910, 505–7.

86. See, for example, "The American Disease," *American Review of Reviews*, October 1905, 497–98; "Great Riches and Sanity," *Outlook*, August 24, 1907, 850–51.

87. William S. Sadler, "Stop a Minute!" *American Magazine*, April 1925, 46–47, 179–83, quote from 46. The term "Americanitis" had appeared earlier. See, for example, Annie Payson Call, *Power through Repose* (Boston: Roberts Brothers, 1891).

88. See, for example, Louis E. Bisch, "Wanted: More Neurotics," *American Mercury*, December 1936, 463–68; Louis E. Bisch, *Be Glad You're Neurotic* (New York: Whittlesey House, 1936).

89. See, for example, Allan McLane Hamilton, "Psychopathic Rulers," *North American Review* (March 1908): 379–87; H. M. Parker, "What Is the Matter with the Kaiser? Insanity Experts Answer the Question," *Illustrated World*, November 1918, 345–48, 468; "The Need of Rational Thinking," *Independent*, May 26, 1923, 330; "Hitler and His Gang," *Living Age*, July 1933, 419–22.

90. "The Delusion of the Crank," *New Republic*, July 10, 1915, 242–43, quote from 243. See also Allan McLane Hamilton, "The Legal Safeguards of Sanity and the Protection of the Insane," *North American Review*, February 1901, 241–49.

91. See, for example, "Insanity in the Army," *Current Literature*, February 1901, 162; "Increasing Insanity," *Current Literature*, May 1904, 547–48; R. L. Duffus, "Is Civilization Driving Us Crazy?" *Scribner's Magazine*, June 1932, 350–52; "Insanity Zones," *Time*, August 17, 1942, 58–60.

92. See, for example, J. Bishop Tingle, "Insanity and Heredity," *Independent*, June 15, 1911, 1305–6; Burton Chance, "Needed Reforms in the Care of the Insane," *Outlook*, December 24, 1904, 1031–38; "Immigration and Insanity," *Hearst's Magazine*, June 1913, 960–61.

93. See, for example, H. H. McClellan, "The Most Neglected People," *Commonweal*, September 18, 1936, 482–83; "Communications: The Most Neglected People," *Commonweal*, October 16, 1936, 584–85; Paul O. Komora, "Not Altogether Neglected," *Commonweal*, December 18, 1936, 207–9; Albert Q. Maisel, "Bedlam 1946," *Life*, May 6, 1946, 102–18.

94. Paul de Kruif, "Men Fixing Life," *Ladies' Home Journal*, June 1932, 18, 117, quote from 117.

95. See, for example, "Chemical Cure for Insanity," *Literary Digest*, November 21, 1931, 16; Wingate M. Johnson, "A New Theory of Insanity," *American Mercury*, January 1933, 64–67; "Radium Treatment for Insanity," *Literary Digest*, May 6, 1933, 21.

96. For early descriptions of treatments for insanity, see, for example, "Water to Quench the Fires of Mania," *Literary Digest*, December 6, 1913, 1109–10.

97. See, for example, "The Brain of Jo Ann," *Newsweek*, April 24, 1944, 28–29. On the changes in the meanings of the diagnosis of schizophrenia over time, see Sander L. Gilman, "Constructing Schizophrenia as a Category of Mental Illness," in Wallace and Gach, *History of Psychiatry and Medical Psychology*, 461–83.

98. C. Charles Burlingame, "Insanity and Insulin," *Forum*, February 1938, 98–102.

99. Greer Williams, "The 'Ex-Insane' Revolt," *Forum*, July 1939, 12–17, quote from 12.

100. See, for example, Albert Deutsch, *The Shame of the States* (New York: Harcourt, Brace, 1948).

101. For an example of the grand claims of psychiatrists in this time period, see, for example, William C. Menninger, "The Role of Psychiatry in the World Today," *American Journal of Psychiatry* 104 (1947): 155–63.

102. For more on the cultural history of anxiety, particularly medications for its treatment, see Andrea Tone, "Listening to the Past: History, Psychiatry, and Anxiety," *Canadian Journal of Psychiatry* 50 (2005): 373–80; Andrea Tone, *The Age of Anxiety: A History of America's Turbulent Affair with Tranquilizers* (New York: Basic Books, 2008).

Chapter 2 — The Expanding Diagnosis of Depression

1. Jonathan O. Cole, "Depression," *American Journal of Psychiatry* 131 (1974): 204–5, quote from 204.

2. David Healy, *The Antidepressant Era* (Cambridge, Mass.: Harvard University Press, 1997).

3. For an excellent, brief social history account of medication development in post–World War II America, see Ruth Schwartz Cowan, *A Social History of American Technology* (New York: Oxford University Press, 1997), 310–25. On the history of the pharmaceutical industry and its relationship to medicine, see Jonathan Liebenau, *Medical Science and Medical Industry: The Formation of the American Pharmaceutical Industry* (Baltimore: Johns Hopkins University Press, 1987); Louis Galambos and Jane Eliot Sewell, *Networks of Innovation: Vaccine Development at Merck, Sharp and Dohme, and Mulford, 1895–1995* (New York: Cambridge University Press, 1995); Peter Temin, *Taking Your Medicine: Drug Regulation in the United States* (Cambridge, Mass.: Harvard University Press, 1980).

4. On the history of psychiatric medications in general, see David Healy, *The Creation of Psychopharmacology* (Cambridge, Mass.: Harvard University Press, 2002). See also Nicolas Rasmussen, "The Drug Industry and Clinical Research in Interwar America: Three Types of Physician Collaborator," *Bulletin of the History of Medicine*

79 (2005): 50–80. For public criticism of psychiatric hospitals in this time period, see chapter 1.

5. Grob, *From Asylum to Community*, 70–92.

6. During this time period, ECT was accepted by virtually all the authors in the psychiatric literature as the definitive treatment for a variety of ailments. The success of medication in helping patients to avoid ECT was frequently mentioned in the 1950s and 1960s. See, for example, Benjamin Pollock, "Clinical Findings in the Use of Tofranil in Depressive and Other Psychiatric States," *American Journal of Psychiatry* 116 (1959): 312–17; David C. English, "A Comparative Study of Antidepressants in Balanced Therapy," *American Journal of Psychiatry* 117 (1961): 865–72; William A. Horwitz, "Physiologic Responses as Prognostic Guides in the Use of Antidepressant Drugs," *American Journal of Psychiatry* 125 (1968): 60–68. On the importance of discharge from the hospital as an outcome measure in this time period, see William F. Orr, Ruth B. Anderson, Margaret Martin, and Des. F. Philpot, "Factors Influencing Discharge of Female Patients from a State Mental Hospital," *American Journal of Psychiatry* 111 (1955): 576–82. On the history of psychiatrists' research with somatic therapies, see Gerald N. Grob, *The Mad among Us: A History of the Care of America's Mentally Ill* (Cambridge, Mass.: Harvard University Press, 1994), 183–89. On the history of ECT, see Shorter and Healy, *Shock Therapy*.

7. See, for example, Herman C. B. Denber and Etta G. Bird, "Chlorpromazine in the Treatment of Mental Illness. III: The Problem of Depression," *American Journal of Psychiatry* 112 (1956): 1021; Joseph A. Barsa and Nathan S. Kline, "Depression Treated with Chlorpromazine and Promethazine," *American Journal of Psychiatry* 113 (1957): 744–45.

8. Jonas B. Robitscher and Sydney E. Pulver, "Orphenadrine in the Treatment of Depression: A Preliminary Study," *American Journal of Psychiatry* 114 (1958): 113–15.

9. See, for example, Frederick Lemere and James H. Lasater, "Deanol (Deaner) a New Cerebral Stimulant for the Treatment of Neurasthenia and Mild Depression: A Preliminary Report," *American Journal of Psychiatry* 114 (1958): 655–56. The idea of using stimulants to combat depression continued to have appeal into the 1970s, when researchers tried methylphenidate and even cocaine. See Ralph N. Wharton, James M. Perel, Peter G. Dayton, and Sidney Malitz, "A Potential Clinical Use for Methylphenidate with Tricyclic Antidepressants," *American Journal of Psychiatry* 127 (1971): 1619–25; Robert M. Post, Joel Kotin, and Frederick K. Goodwin, "The Effects of Cocaine on Depressed Patients," *American Journal of Psychiatry* 131 (1974): 511–17. Rasmussen has pointed out that stimulants were used and marketed in an outpatient setting decades earlier. Rasmussen, "Making the First Anti-Depressant"; Rasmussen, *On Speed*.

10. After the apparent success of iproniazid, some researchers tried out other antituberculosis medications to see if they would help with depressive states. See, for example, George E. Crane, "Cyloserine as an Antidepressant Agent," *American Journal of Psychiatry* 115 (1959): 1025–26.

11. See, for example, Antonio J. DeLiz Ferreira and Harry Freeman, "A Clinical Trial of Marsilid in Psychotic Depressed Patients," *American Journal of Psychiatry* 114 (1958): 933–34.

12. For an example of improvement in outpatients on an antidepressant "stimulating" agent, see Howard D. Fabing, J. Robert Hawkins, and James A. L. Moulton, "Clinical Studies on a-(2-Piperidyl) Benzhydrol Hydrochloride, a New Antidepressant Drug," *American Journal of Psychiatry* 111 (1955): 832–37.

13. H. Azima and R. H. Vispo, "Imipramine: A Potent New Anti-Depressant Compound," *American Journal of Psychiatry* 115 (1958): 245–46. Roland Kuhn, the researcher credited with the discovery of imipramine, summarized his research in Switzerland in his 1958 review article, "The Treatment of Depressive States with G22355 (Imipramine Hydrochloride)," *American Journal of Psychiatry* 115 (1958): 459–64.

14. Theodore R. Robie, "Iproniazid Chemotherapy in Melancholia," *American Journal of Psychiatry* 115 (1958): 402–9, quote from 407, emphasis added.

15. Pollock, "Clinical Findings in the Use of Tofranil," 314.

16. The issue of consent in psychiatric treatment and research is a large and complicated one, and its history has not been fully explored. Turner in 1962 mentioned that, with the changing demographics of hospital populations by the 1960s and the increasing number of voluntary patients, electroshock therapy declined because voluntary patients would not agree to it. William J. Turner, Francis J. O'Neill, and Sidney Merlis, "The Treatment of Depression in Hospitalized Patients before and since the Introduction of Antidepressant Drugs," *American Journal of Psychiatry* 119 (1962): 421–26. The first incidence I could find of a researcher mentioning that patients signed an informed consent prior to participation in a clinical trial was Sidney Malitz and Maureen Kanzler, "Are Antidepressants Better Than Placebo?" *American Journal of Psychiatry* 127 (1971): 1605–11. For a history of earlier human experimentation, see Susan E. Lederer, *Subjected to Science: Human Experimentation in America before the Second World War* (Baltimore: Johns Hopkins University Press, 1995).

17. For historical analysis of the emergence of clinical trials, see Harry M. Marks, *The Progress of Experiment: Science and Therapeutic Reform in the United States, 1900–1990* (New York: Cambridge University Press, 1997).

18. Robert R. Schopbach, "Clinical Note Concerning Iproniazid (Marsilid)," *American Journal of Psychiatry* 114 (1958): 838–39.

19. Erwin L. Linn, "Sources of Uncertainty in Studies of Drugs Affecting Mood, Mentation or Activity," *American Journal of Psychiatry* 116 (1959): 97–103.

20. See, for example, Norman Roulet et al., "Imipramine in Depression: A Controlled Study," *American Journal of Psychiatry* 119 (1962): 427–31.

21. In addition, researchers sometimes used electroshock therapy as a comparison treatment, although researchers acknowledged that it was not possible to double blind the group receiving shock treatments. Milton Greenblatt, George H. Grosser, and Henry Wechsler, "A Comparative Study of Selected Antidepressant Medications and EST," *American Journal of Psychiatry* 119 (1962): 144–53; Milton Greenblatt, George H. Grosser, and Henry Wechsler, "Differential Response of Hospitalized Depressed Patients to Somatic Therapy," *American Journal of Psychiatry* 120 (1964): 935–43.

22. For examples of the continuing use of case reports and analysis, see Milton Kramer, Roy M. Whitman, Bill Baldridge, and Leonard Lansky, "Depression: Dreams and Defenses," *American Journal of Psychiatry* 122 (1965): 411–19; Milton Kramer, Roy M. Whitman, Bill Baldridge, and Paul H. Ornstein, "Drugs and Dreams III: The Effects of Imipramine on the Dreams of Depressed Patients," *American Journal of Psychiatry* 124 (1968): 1385–92.

23. John Holt, Eleanore R. Wright, and Arthur O. Hecker, "Comparative Clinical Experience with Five Antidepressants," *American Journal of Psychiatry* 117 (1960): 533–38.

24. John E. Overall, Leo E. Hollister, Merlin Johnson, and Veronica Pennington, "Nosology of Depression and Differential Response to Drugs," *Journal of the American Medical Association* 195 (1966): 946–48.

25. Jonathan Metzl has pointed out that psychoanalytic concepts remained embedded in biological approaches to patients. Metzl, *Prozac on the Couch.*

26. Historian Jonathan Sadowsky has explored the importance of links between psychoanalytic and biological perspectives in ECT. Sadowsky, "Beyond the Metaphor of the Pendulum." For an example of a blending of psychoanalysis and medication in practice, see Gerald J. Sarwer-Foner, ed., *The Dynamics of Psychiatric Drug Therapy: A Conference on the Psychodynamic, Psychoanalytic, and Sociologic Aspects of the Neuroleptic Drugs in Psychiatry* (Springfield, Ill.: Thomas, 1960).

27. See, for example, Leo H. Bartemeier, "Presidential Address," *American Journal of Psychiatry* 109 (1952): 1–7; Arthur Noyes, "Presidential Address," *American Journal of Psychiatry* 112 (1955): 1–7; Francis J. Gerty, "The Physician and Psychotherapy," *American Journal of Psychiatry* 116 (1959): 1–10.

28. Walter E. Barton, "Presidential Address: Psychiatry in Transition," *American Journal of Psychiatry* 119 (1962): 1–15, quote from 5. See also C. H. Hardin Branch, "Presidential Address: Preparedness for Progress," *American Journal of Psychiatry* 120 (1963): 1–11.

29. For the possible application of science within a psychoanalytic approach, see, for example, Francis J. Braceland, "Psychiatry and the Science of Man," *American Journal of Psychiatry* 114 (1957): 1–9.

30. Spitzer and Endicott were enormously productive in this area in the 1960s and 1970s, and some of their publications contained similar descriptions intended for different audiences. The citations that follow represent a sample of their work.

31. Robert L. Spitzer, Jean Endicott, and Joseph L. Fleiss, "Instruments and Recording Forms for Evaluating Psychiatric Status and History: Rationale, Method of Development and Description," *Comprehensive Psychiatry* 8 (1967): 321–43, quote from 325.

32. On his admission about his psychoanalytic training, see, for example, Robert L. Spitzer, "Mental Status Schedule: Potential Use as a Criterion Measure of Change in Psychotherapy Research," *American Journal of Psychotherapy* 20 (1966): 156–67.

33. Patricia Neely Wold and Kirby Dwight, "Subtypes of Depression Identified by the KDS-3A: A Pilot Study," *American Journal of Psychiatry* 136 (1979): 1415–19. See also Brigitte A. Prusoff, Myrna M. Weissman, Gerald L. Klerman, and Bruce J. Rounsaville, "Research Diagnostic Criteria Subtypes of Depression: Their Role as Predictors of Differential Response to Psychotherapy and Drug Treatment," *Archives of General Psychiatry* 37 (1980): 796–801.

34. James J. Cadden and Frederic F. Flach, "Differential Response to Treatment as a Function of the Changing Character of Depression," *American Journal of Psychiatry* 126 (1970): 1013–16.

35. Myer Mendelson, *Psychoanalytic Concepts of Depression* (Springfield, Ill.: Thomas, 1960).

36. Allen Raskin, Joy Schulterbrandt, Natalie Reatig, and James J. McKeon, "Replication of Factors of Psychopathology in Interview, Ward Behavior and Self-Report Ratings of Hospitalized Depressives," *Journal of Nervous and Mental Disease* 148 (1969): 87–98, quote from 87.

37. See, for example, Lino Covi, Ronald S. Lipman, Renato D. Alarcon, and Virginia K. Smith, "Drug and Psychotherapy Interactions in Depression," *American Journal of Psychiatry* 133 (1976): 502–8.

38. David R. Hawkins and Joseph Mendels, "Sleep Disturbance in Depressive Syndromes," *American Journal of Psychiatry* 123 (1966): 682–700.

39. Robert A. Woodruff Jr., George E. Murphy, and Marijan Herjanic, "The Natural History of Affective Disorders—I. Symptoms of 72 Patients at the Time of Index Hospital Admission," *Journal of Psychiatric Research* 5 (1967): 255–63.

40. For a contemporary overview of changes in research over this time period, see H. Keith H. Brodie and Melvin Sabshin, "An Overview of Trends in Psychiatric Research: 1963–1972," *American Journal of Psychiatry* 130 (1973): 1309–18.

41. See, for example, Arthur J. Prange et al., "Enhancement of Imipramine by Thyroid Stimulating Hormone: Clinical and Theoretical Implications," *American Journal of Psychiatry* 127 (1970): 191–99; Karl Rickels et al., "Amitriptyline and Trimipramine in Neurotic Depressed Outpatients: A Collaborative Study," *American Journal of Psychiatry* 127 (1970): 208–18; Robert V. DeSilverio et al., "Perphenazine-Amitriptyline in Neurotic Depressed Outpatients: A Controlled Collaborative Study," *American Journal of Psychiatry* 127 (1970): 322–28; Karl Rickels et al., "Amitriptyline in Anxious-Depressed Outpatients: A Controlled Study," *American Journal of Psychiatry* 131 (1974): 25–30; Allen Raskin, "A Guide for Drug Use in Depressive Disorders," *American Journal of Psychiatry* 131 (1974): 181–85.

42. For contemporary explanations of the group, see Martin M. Katz and Gerald L. Klerman, "Introduction: Overview of the Clinical Studies Program," *American Journal of Psychiatry* 136 (1979): 49–51; Martin M. Katz, Steven K. Secunda, Robert M. A. Hirschfeld, and Stephen H. Koslow, "NIMH Clinical Research Branch Collaborative Program on the Psychobiology of Depression," *Archives of General Psychiatry* 36 (1979): 765–71. For a retrospective account of the group, see Morris B. Parloff and Irene Elkin, "The NIMH Treatment of Depression Collaborative Research Program," in *History of Psychotherapy: A Century of Change*, ed. Donald K. Freedheim (Washington, D.C.: American Psychological Association, 1992), 442–49. For a history of psychiatric and neuroscience activities at the National Institutes of Health (NIH), see Ingrid G. Farreras, Caroline Hannaway, and Victoria A. Harden, eds., *Mind, Brain, Body, and Behavior: Foundations of Neuroscience and Behavioral Research at the National Institutes of Health* (Washington, D.C.: IOS Press, 2004).

43. Katz et al., "NIMH Clinical Research Branch Collaborative Program."

44. Katz and Klerman, "Introduction," 49.

45. The first study that I found that was sponsored (including study design and statistical analysis) by a pharmaceutical company (Geigy) was Abraham Heller, Rorry Zahourek, and H. G. Whittington, "Effectiveness of Antidepressant Drugs: A Triple-Blind Study Comparing Imipramine, Desipramine, and Placebo," *American Journal of Psychiatry* 127 (1971): 1092–95. See also the Australian study, A. Kessell, T. A. A. Pearce, and N. F. Holt, "A Controlled Study of Nortriptyline and Imipramine," *American Journal of Psychiatry* 126 (1970): 938–45. The current pharmaceutical industry role in clinical research is a subject of intense discussion and disagreement. See, for example, Healy, *Let Them Eat Prozac*.

46. David Healy, "Manufacturing Consensus," *Culture, Medicine & Psychiatry* 30 (2006): 135–56.

47. See, for example, Helmut Beckmann and Frederick K. Goodwin, "Antidepressant Response to Tricyclics and Urinary MHPG in Unipolar Patients: Clinical Response to Imipramine or Amitriptyline," *Archives of General Psychiatry* 32 (1975): 17–21.

48. See, for example, John Feighner et al., "Hormonal Potentiation of Imipramine and ECT in Primary Depression," *American Journal of Psychiatry* 128 (1972): 1230–38.

49. See, for example, Anthony LaPolla and Harry Jones, "Placebo-Control Evaluation of Desipramine in Depression," *American Journal of Psychiatry* 127 (1970): 335–38.

50. Maria Kovacs, "The Efficacy of Cognitive and Behavior Therapies for Depression," *American Journal of Psychiatry* 137 (1980): 1495–1501.

51. Aaron T. Beck, *Cognitive Therapy and the Emotional Disorders* (New York: International Universities Press, 1976).

52. For the latest version of Interpersonal Psychotherapy, see Myrna M. Weissman, John C. Markowitz, and Gerald L. Klerman, *Comprehensive Guide to Interpersonal Psychotherapy* (New York: Basic Books, 2000).

53. Myrna M. Weissman, "The Psychological Treatment of Depression: Evidence for the Efficacy of Psychotherapy Alone, in Comparison with, and in Combination with Pharmacotherapy," *Archives of General Psychiatry* 36 (1979): 1261–69, quote from 1268.

54. Gerald N. Grob, "Origins of *DSM-I*: A Study in Appearance and Reality," *American Journal of Psychiatry* 148 (1991): 421–30; American Psychiatric Association, *Diagnostic and Statistical Manual: Mental Disorders* (Washington, D.C.: American Psychiatric Association, 1952).

55. Marvin Brandwin, an associate of Moses Frohlich—one of the chairmen of the APA Committee on Nomenclature and Statistics—prepared a report for Frohlich in 1956 that suggested that national criticism of the first edition of the *DSM* was relatively minor and mostly related to codes and usage. "Report on Diagnostic Manual," personal papers of Marvin Brandwin, Ann Arbor, Mich. (used by permission).

56. See, for example, Aaron T. Beck, "Reliability of Psychiatric Diagnoses: 1. A Critique of Systematic Studies," *American Journal of Psychiatry* 119 (1962): 210–16.

57. In 1967, Spitzer quantified reliability by adapting a statistic known as the kappa coefficient, originally defined in a 1960 publication on general biometric measures, for use in assessing psychiatric diagnosis. See Robert L. Spitzer, Jacob Cohen, Joseph L. Fleiss, and Jean Endicott, "Quantification of Agreement in Psychiatric Diagnosis: A New Approach," *Archives of General Psychiatry* 17 (1967): 83–87; Jacob Cohen, "A Coefficient of Agreement for Nominal Scales," *Educational and Psychological Measurement* 20 (1960): 37–46.

58. For a clear explanation of Spitzer and the reliability issue, see Stuart A. Kirk and Herb Kutchins, *The Selling of DSM: The Rhetoric of Science in Psychiatry* (New York: Aldine de Gruyter, 1992); Herb Kutchins and Stuart A. Kirk, *Making Us Crazy: DSM, The Psychiatric Bible and the Creation of Mental Disorders* (New York: Free Press, 1997).

59. Psychiatrists who were enthusiastic about diagnosis and statistics had actually started using punch cards for electronic record keeping as early as the 1930s. See, for example, Neil A. Dayton, "The New Statistical System of the Massachusetts Department of Mental Diseases," *American Journal of Psychiatry* 86 (1930): 779–803.

60. Jean Endicott reported that the attempt to use computer modeling with *DSM-II* diagnoses illustrated the subjective and often illogical ways in which psychiatrists made diagnoses. Jean Endicott, "Severe Premenstrual Syndrome: From No Diagnosis or Treatment to Multiple Treatments," Grand Rounds, University of Michigan Department of Psychiatry, November 2, 2005, Ann Arbor. On the computer simulations, see Robert L. Spitzer and Loretta M. Gilford, "UPDATE: A Computer Program for Converting Diagnoses to the New Nomenclature of the American Psychiatric Association," *American Journal of Psychiatry* 125 (1968): 395–96; Robert L. Spitzer and Jean Endicott, "DIAGNO: A Computer Program for Psychiatric Diagnosis Utilizing the Differential Diagnostic Procedure," *Archives of General Psychiatry* 18 (1968):

746–56; Robert L. Spitzer and Jean Endicott, "DIAGNO II: Further Developments in a Computer Program for Psychiatric Diagnosis," *American Journal of Psychiatry* 125, Supp. (1969): 112–21.

61. Walter E. Barton, "Prospects and Perspectives: Implications of Social Change for Psychiatry," *American Journal of Psychiatry* 125 (1968): 147–50, quote from 147.

62. In the late 1950s, Thomas Szasz, in an article in the *American Journal of Psychiatry*, began a critique of the disease model of mental disorders implied by a classification scheme. Szasz eventually developed this critique into his influential argument that mental illness was a myth. Thomas S. Szasz, "The Problem of Psychiatric Nosology: A Contribution to a Situational Analysis of Psychiatric Operations," *American Journal of Psychiatry* 114 (1957): 405–13; Thomas S. Szasz, "The Myth of Mental Illness," *American Psychologist* 15 (1960): 113–18. See Richard E. Vatz and Lee S. Weinberg, "The Rhetorical Paradigm in Psychiatric History: Thomas Szasz and the Myth of Mental Illness," in *Discovering the History of Psychiatry*, ed. Mark S. Micale and Roy Porter (New York: Oxford University Press, 1994), 311–30.

63. See, for example, Bertram S. Brown, "Psychiatric Practice and Public Policy," *American Journal of Psychiatry* 125 (1968): 141–46.

64. *DSM-II* is perhaps best known for being the edition in which homosexuality appeared as a diagnosis, then disappeared in 1973 after a contentious APA vote. See Bayer, *Homosexuality and American Psychiatry*.

65. See copyright page, American Psychiatric Association, *Diagnostic and Statistical Manual of Mental Disorders*, 2nd ed. (Washington, D.C.: American Psychiatric Association, 1968).

66. See, for example, Robert L. Spitzer, "A Response to the Threat of a Classification Scheme for the Psychosocial Disorders: Some Specific Suggestions," *American Journal of Orthopsychiatry* 41 (1971): 838–40. Spitzer was not alone in his complaints about the deficiencies in *DSM-II*. See, for example, Martin M. Katz, Jonathan O. Cole, and Henri A. Lowery, "Studies of the Diagnostic Process: The Influence of Symptom Perception, Past Experience, and Ethnic Background on Diagnostic Decisions," *American Journal of Psychiatry* 125 (1969): 937–47; Basil Jackson, "The Revised Diagnostic and Statistical Manual of the American Psychiatric Association," *American Journal of Psychiatry* 127 (1970): 65–73.

67. John Feighner et al., "Diagnostic Criteria for Use in Psychiatric Research," *Archives of General Psychiatry* 26 (1972): 57–63.

68. Joseph L. Fleiss, Robert L. Spitzer, Jean Endicott, and Jacob Cohen, "Quantification of Agreement in Multiple Psychiatric Diagnosis," *Archives of General Psychiatry* 26 (1972): 168–71, quote from 168.

69. See Robert L. Spitzer, Jean Endicott, and Eli Robins, "Research Diagnostic Criteria," *Psychopharmacology Bulletin* 11 (1975): 22–25; Robert L. Spitzer, Jean Endicott, and Eli Robins, "Research Diagnostic Criteria: Rationale and Reliability," *Archives of General Psychiatry* 35 (1978): 773–82; Robert L. Spitzer, Jean Endicott, and Janet B. W. Williams, "Research Diagnostic Criteria," *Archives of General Psychiatry* 36 (1979): 1381–83.

70. Jean Endicott and Robert L. Spitzer, "Use of the Research Diagnostic Criteria and the Schedule for Affective Disorders and Schizophrenia to Study Affective Disorders," *American Journal of Psychiatry* 136 (1979): 52–56.

71. See, for example, Robert S. Garber, "The Presidential Address: The Proper Business of Psychiatry," *American Journal of Psychiatry* 128 (1971): 1–11; John Spiegel,

"Response to the Presidential Address," *American Journal of Psychiatry* 131 (1974): 754–56.

72. Judd Marmor, "Response to the Presidential Address," *American Journal of Psychiatry* 132 (1975): 698–99; Jules H. Masserman, "Response to the Presidential Address," *American Journal of Psychiatry* 135 (1978): 900–903.

73. See Robert L. Spitzer, Janet B. W. Williams, and Andrew E. Skodol, "*DSM-III*: The Major Achievements and an Overview," *American Journal of Psychiatry* 137 (1980): 151–64; Ronald Bayer and Robert L. Spitzer, "Neurosis, Psychodynamics, and *DSM-III*: A History of the Controversy," *Archives of General Psychiatry* 42 (1985): 187–96.

74. Mitchell Wilson, "DSM-III and the Transformation of American Psychiatry: A History," *American Journal of Psychiatry* 150 (1993): 399–410.

75. Spitzer had work groups for a number of major diagnostic groups. *DSM* Collection, Robert L. Spitzer Papers, Melvin Sabshin Library and Archives, American Psychiatric Association, Washington, D.C.

76. Depression Folder, *DSM* Collection, Box 2, Spitzer Papers.

77. Cover letter for questionnaire by Robert Spitzer, May 18, 1978, Depression Folder, *DSM* Collection, Box 2, Spitzer Papers.

78. Gerald L. Klerman, Jean Endicott, Robert L. Spitzer, and Robert M. A. Hirschfeld, "Neurotic Depressions: A Systematic Analysis of Multiple Criteria and Meanings," *American Journal of Psychiatry* 136 (1979): 57–61.

79. See Paula Clayton to Spitzer, February 9, 1979; E. H. Uhlenhuth to Spitzer, February 13, 1979; Bernard Carroll to Spitzer, February 19, 1979, all in Depression Folder, *DSM* Collection, Box 2, Spitzer Papers.

80. Nancy C. Andreasen and George Winokur, "Secondary Depression: Familial, Clinical, and Research Perspectives," *American Journal of Psychiatry* 136 (1979): 62–66, quote from 62. See also George Winokur, "Unipolar Depression: Is It Divisible Into Autonomous Subtypes?" *Archives of General Psychiatry* 36 (1979): 47–52; Nancy Andreasen and George Winokur, "Newer Experimental Methods for Classifying Depression," *Archives of General Psychiatry* 36 (1979): 447–52.

81. In the *DSM-III* descriptions of depression, there was a modifier, "With Melancholia," which consisted of worsening depression in the morning, early morning awakening, weight loss, and inappropriate guilt. American Psychiatric Association, *Diagnostic and Statistical Manual of Mental Disorders*, 3rd ed., 215. It is not clear that this modifier was used much, however.

82. American Psychiatric Association, *Diagnostic and Statistical Manual of Mental Disorders*, 3rd ed., 205–24.

83. See, for example, Andrew E. Skodol, Robert L. Spitzer, and Janet B. W. Williams, "Teaching and Learning DSM-III," *American Journal of Psychiatry* 138 (1981): 1581–86.

84. See Mood Folders, *DSM* Collection, Spitzer Papers.

85. American Psychiatric Association, *Diagnostic and Statistical Manual of Mental Disorders*, 3rd rev. ed. (Washington, D.C.: American Psychiatric Press, 1987), 222–24, quote from 224. See also Mark Zimmerman and Robert L. Spitzer, "Melancholia: From DSM-III to DSM-III-R," *American Journal of Psychiatry* 146 (1989): 20–28. It is not clear whether the melancholia subtype was actually used in clinical practice.

86. The debate around categorical diagnoses has gained new energy in recent years in anticipation of *DSM-V*, especially in the area of personality disorders. See, for example, Thomas A. Widiger, Erik Simonsen, Paul J. Sirovatka, and Darrel A. Regier,

eds., *Dimensional Models of Personality Disorders: Refining the Research Agenda for DSM-V* (Washington, D.C.: American Psychiatric Association Press, 2006). For the official statements on *DSM-V* plans, see David J. Kupfer, Michael B. First, and Darrel A. Regier, eds., *A Research Agenda for DSM-V* (Washington, D.C.: American Psychiatric Association Press, 2002).

87. T. R. Robie, "Marsilid in Depression," *American Journal of Psychiatry* 114 (1958): 936–37.

88. Joseph J. Schildkraut, "The Catecholamine Hypothesis of Affective Disorders: A Review of Supporting Evidence," *American Journal of Psychiatry* 122 (1965): 509–22, quote from 509. See also Joseph J. Schildkraut, Saul M. Schanberg, George R. Breese, and Irwin J. Kopin, "Norepinephrine Metabolism and Drugs Used in the Affective Disorders: A Possible Mechanism of Action," *American Journal of Psychiatry* 124 (1967): 600–608; Joseph A. Schildkraut, "Norepinephrine Metabolites as Biochemical Criteria for Classifying Depressive Disorders and Predicting Responses to Treatment: Preliminary Findings," *American Journal of Psychiatry* 130 (1973): 695–99.

89. Schildkraut's hypothesis has remained compelling, though the evidence has not been as supportive as investigators originally hoped. See, for example, David L. Dunner and Ronald R. Fieve, "Affective Disorder: Studies with Amine Precursors," *American Journal of Psychiatry* 132 (1975): 180–83; Joe Mendels, James L. Stinnett, David Burns, and Alan Frazer, "Amine Precursors and Depression," *Archives of General Psychiatry* 32 (1975): 22–30. A 1985 reformulation of the hypothesis put it in terms of homeostasis in the mode of Claude Bernard. Larry J. Siever and Kenneth L. Davis, "Overview: Toward a Dysregulation Hypothesis of Depression," *American Journal of Psychiatry* 142 (1985): 1017–31.

90. A similar process of inferring backward from drug effect occurred in schizophrenia. Researchers in the 1960s and 1970s concluded that since chlorpromazine seemed to help in schizophrenia and since the medication reduced dopamine, schizophrenia was caused by abnormal dopamine levels. This hypothesis has been seriously questioned in recent years, however.

91. Anthony M. D'Agostino, "Depression: Schism in Contemporary Psychiatry," *American Journal of Psychiatry* 132 (1975): 629–32, quote from 629.

92. Donald F. Klein, "Endogenomorphic Depression: A Conceptual and Terminological Revision," *Archives of General Psychiatry* 31 (1974): 447–54; Hagop S. Akiskal and William T. McKinney Jr., "Overview of Recent Research in Depression: Integration of Ten Conceptual Models into a Comprehensive Clinical Frame," *Archives of General Psychiatry* 32 (1975): 285–305.

93. See, for example, Frank DeLeon-Jones, James W. Maas, Haroutune Dekirmenjian, and Jesus Sanchez, "Diagnostic Subgroups of Affective Disorders and Their Urinary Excretion of Catecholamine Metabolites," *American Journal of Psychiatry* 132 (1975): 1141–48; Duane G. Spiker et al., "Urinary MHPG and Clinical Response to Amitriptyline in Depressed Patients," *American Journal of Psychiatry* 137 (1980): 1183–87; Giovanni Muscettola et al., "Imipramine and Desipramine in Plasma and Spinal Fluid," *Archives of General Psychiatry* 35 (1978): 621–25.

94. Paul E. Garfinkel, Jerry J. Warsh, and Harvey C. Stancer, "Depression: New Evidence in Support of Biological Differentiation," *American Journal of Psychiatry* 136 (1979): 535–39.

95. See, for example, Jonathan R. T. Davidson et al., "Platelet Monoamine Oxidase Activity and the Classification of Depression," *Archives of General Psychiatry*

37 (1980): 771–73; Jon E. Gudeman et al., "Toward a Biochemical Classification of Depressive Disorders, VI: Platelet MAO Activity and Clinical Symptoms in Depressed Patients," *American Journal of Psychiatry* 139 (1982): 630–33. MAOIs were (and remain) somewhat difficult to use. When patients take MAOIs, they are required to be on a special diet, which excludes aged cheese, wine, and other tyromine-heavy foods. Ingestion of these foods could lead to dangerously high blood pressure and possibly even death.

96. For a longer view on medical interest in stress hormones, see Harry M. Marks, "Cortisone, 1949: A Year in the Political Life of a Drug," *Bulletin of the History of Medicine* 66 (1992): 419–39.

97. Bernard J. Carroll et al., "Plasma Dexamethasone Concentrations and Cortisol Suppression Response in Patients with Endogenous Depression," *Journal of Clinical Endocrinology and Metabolism* 51 (1980): 433–37.

98. See, for example, Walter Armin Brown, Robert Johnston, and Demmie Mayfield, "The 24-Hour Dexamethasone Suppression Test in a Clinical Setting: Relationship to Diagnosis, Symptoms, and Response to Treatment," *American Journal of Psychiatry* 136 (1979): 543–47.

99. Kenneth L. Davis et al., "Neuroendocrine and Neurochemical Measurements in Depression," *American Journal of Psychiatry* 138 (1981): 1555–62, quote from 1555.

100. The other medical specialty that led the way in terms of medical technology was cardiology. See Kirk Jeffrey, *Machines in Our Hearts: The Cardiac Pacemaker, the Implantable Defibrillator, and American Health Care* (Baltimore: Johns Hopkins University Press, 2001). For historical perspective on the increasing technologies around the human body in the second half of the century, see David Serlin, *Replaceable You: Engineering the Body in Postwar America* (Chicago: University of Chicago Press, 2004).

101. By this time, the older application of heredity in medicine—eugenics—had been largely stripped of its political overtones and refashioned as genetics. See Diane B. Paul, "From Eugenics to Medical Genetics," *Journal of Policy History* 9 (1997): 96–116; Diane B. Paul, *Controlling Human Heredity, 1865 to the Present* (Atlantic Highlands, N.J.: Humanities Press, 1995); Kevles, *In the Name of Eugenics*; Kenneth M. Ludmerer, *Genetics and American Society: A Historical Appraisal* (Baltimore: Johns Hopkins University Press, 1972).

102. George Winokur, "Familial (Genetic) Subtypes of Pure Depressive Disease," *American Journal of Psychiatry* 136 (1979): 911–13.

103. Winokur, "Unipolar Depression."

104. Silvano Arieti and Jules R. Bemporad, "The Psychological Organization of Depression," *American Journal of Psychiatry* 137 (1980): 1360–65, quote from 1360; Silvano Arieti, "Psychotherapy of Severe Depression," *American Journal of Psychiatry* 134 (1977): 864–68.

105. For calls for biological (primarily in terms of research and medications) emphasis within psychiatry, see, for example, Daniel X. Freedman, "Presidential Address: Science in the Service of the Ill," *American Journal of Psychiatry* 139 (1982): 1087–95; H. Keith H. Brodie, "Presidential Address: Psychiatry—Its Locus and Its Future," *American Journal of Psychiatry* 140 (1983): 965–68.

106. See, for example, John M. Davis, "Overview: Maintenance Therapy in Psychiatry: II. Affective Disorders," *American Journal of Psychiatry* 133 (1976): 1–13; David L. Dunner, Frank Stallone, and Ronald R. Fieve, "Lithium Carbonate and Affective

Disorders," *Archives of General Psychiatry* 33 (1976): 117–20; Robert F. Prien, C. James Klett, and Eugene M. Caffey Jr., "Lithium Prophylaxis in Recurrent Affective Illness," *American Journal of Psychiatry* 131 (1974): 198–203. One of the most enthusiastic proponents of lithium treatment was Ronald Fieve at the New York State Psychiatric Institute. See, for example, Ronald R. Fieve, Stanley R. Platman, and Robert R. Plutchik, "The Use of Lithium in Affective Disorders: I. Acute Endogenous Depression," *American Journal of Psychiatry* 125 (1968): 487–91; Ronald R. Fieve, Stanley R. Platman, and Robert R. Plutchik, "The Use of Lithium in Affective Disorders: II. Prophylaxis of Depression in Chronic Recurrent Affective Disorder," *American Journal of Psychiatry* 125 (1968): 492–98; Robert R. Fieve, Turkan Kumbaraci, and David L. Dunner, "Lithium Prophylaxis of Depression in Bipolar I, Bipolar II, and Unipolar Patients," *American Journal of Psychiatry* 133 (1976): 925–29.

107. See, for example, Thomas J. Craig and Pearl A. Van Natta, "Presence and Persistence of Depressive Symptoms in Patient and Community Populations," *American Journal of Psychiatry* 133 (1976): 1426–29; George W. Comstock and Knud J. Helsing, "Symptoms of Depression in Two Communities," *Psychological Medicine* 6 (1976): 551–63; Myrna M. Weissman et al., "Assessing Depressive Symptoms in Five Psychiatric Populations: A Validation Study," *American Journal of Epidemiology* 106 (1977): 203–14.

108. For shifts in disease epidemiology from acute to chronic disease in the second half of the twentieth century, see Daniel M. Fox, "Health Policy and Changing Epidemiology in the United States: Chronic Disease in the Twentieth Century," *Transactions and Studies of the College of Physicians of Philadelphia* 10 (1988): 11–31.

109. Charlotte Silverman, "The Epidemiology of Depression—A Review," *American Journal of Psychiatry* 124 (1968): 883–91.

110. Lee N. Robins, John E. Helzer, Jack Croughan, and Kathryn S. Ratcliff, "National Institute of Mental Health Diagnostic Interview Schedule: Its History, Characteristics, and Validity," *Archives of General Psychiatry* 38 (1981): 381–89.

111. In 1969, Morton Kramer noted that the rates of admission for schizophrenia were substantially higher in the United States than in England, likely because of differences in diagnostic methodology. Morton Kramer, "Cross-National Study of Diagnosis of the Mental Disorders," *American Journal of Psychiatry* 125, Supp. (1969): 1–11.

112. Darrel A. Regier et al., "One-Month Prevalence of Mental Disorders in the United States: Based on Five Epidemiologic Catchment Area Sites," *Archives of General Psychiatry* 45 (1988): 977–86.

113. For U.S. psychiatrists' efforts to educate primary care physicians about depression, see, for example, Remi J. Cadoret, Reuben B. Widmer, and Carol North, "Depression in Family Practice: Long-Term Prognosis and Somatic Complaints," *Journal of Family Practice* 10 (1980): 625–29; Michael J. Garvey, "Biochemistry and Treatment Strategies for Depression," *Journal of Family Practice* 11 (1980): 215–19. For a historical perspective on this issue, see Christopher M. Callahan and German E. Berrios, *Reinventing Depression: A History of the Treatment of Depression in Primary Care, 1940–2004* (New York: Oxford University Press, 2005).

114. See, for example, Aaron T. Beck and Alice Beamesderfer, "Assessment of Depression: The Depression Inventory," *Modern Problems of Pharmacopsychiatry* 7 (1974): 151–69. For more discussion of the origins and content of the Beck Depression Inventory (BDI), see chapter 4.

115. Sidney Zisook, Richard C. W. Hall, and Elizabeth Gammon, "Drug Treatment of Depression: A Classification System for Agent Selection," *Postgraduate Medicine* 67 (1980): 153–61, quote from 153.
116. Martin B. Keller et al., "Treatment Received by Depressed Patients," *Journal of the American Medical Association* 248 (1982): 1848–55.
117. See, for example, Reuben B. Widmer and Remi J. Cadoret, "Depression: The Great Imitator in Family Practice," *Journal of Family Practice* 17 (1983): 485–86, 495–98, 503–5.
118. See, for example, Consensus Development Panel, "Mood Disorders: Pharmacologic Prevention of Recurrences," *American Journal of Psychiatry* 142 (1985): 469–76; Martin B. Keller, "Undertreatment of Major Depression," *Psychopharmacology Bulletin* 24 (1988): 75–80.
119. Martin B. Keller and Robert W. Shapiro, "'Double Depression': Superimposition of Acute Depressive Episodes on Chronic Depressive Disorders," *American Journal of Psychiatry* 139 (1982): 438–42. See also Martin B. Keller et al., "'Double Depression': Two-Year Follow-Up," *American Journal of Psychiatry* 140 (1983): 689–94.
120. Marsha K. Stein, Karl Rickels, and Charles C. Weise, "Maintenance Therapy with Amitriptyline: A Controlled Trial," *American Journal of Psychiatry* 137 (1980): 370–71.
121. Robert W. Shapiro and Martin B. Keller, "Initial 6-Month Follow-Up of Patients with Major Depressive Disorder," *Journal of Affective Disorders* 3 (1981): 205–20.
122. Martin B. Keller and Robert W. Shapiro, "Major Depressive Disorder: Initial Results from a One-Year Prospective Naturalistic Follow-Up Study," *Journal of Nervous and Mental Disease* 169 (1981): 761–68.
123. Martin B. Keller, Philip W. Lavori, Collins E. Lewis, and Gerald L. Klerman, "Predictors of Relapse in Major Depressive Disorder," *Journal of the American Medical Association* 250 (1983): 3299–3304; Robert F. Prien and David J. Kupfer, "Continuation Drug Therapy for Major Depressive Episodes: How Long Should It Be Maintained?" *American Journal of Psychiatry* 143 (1986): 18–23; David J. Kupfer and Ellen Frank, "Relapse in Recurrent Unipolar Depression," *American Journal of Psychiatry* 144 (1987): 86–88.
124. Consensus Development Panel, "Mood Disorders," 472.
125. Darrel A. Regier et al., "The NIMH Depression Awareness, Recognition, and Treatment Program: Structure, Aims, and Scientific Basis," *American Journal of Psychiatry* 145 (1988): 1351–57.
126. Myrna M. Weissman, Stanislav V. Kasl, and Gerald L. Klerman, "Follow-Up of Depressed Women after Maintenance Treatment," *American Journal of Psychiatry* 133 (1976): 757–60, quote from 760.
127. A number of historians have pointed out the importance of shifting federal support for research and treatment of chronic diseases in the twentieth century. See, for example, Steven J. Peitzman, "From Bright's Disease to End-Stage Renal Disease," in Rosenberg and Golden, *Framing Disease*, 3–19; Fox, "Health Policy."
128. Alan Stoudemire et al., "The Economic Burden of Depression," *General Hospital Psychiatry* 8 (1986): 387–94.
129. David Healy, "The Intersection of Psychopharmacology and Psychiatry in the Second Half of the Twentieth Century," in Wallace and Gach, *History of Psychiatry and Medical Psychology*, 419–37.
130. Bayer and Spitzer, "Neurosis, Psychodynamics, and DSM-III."
131. Between 1940 and 1960, the *American Journal of Psychiatry* contained approxi-

mately as many articles on anxiety as on depression. By the 1960s, however, the number of articles on depression became significantly greater than the number on anxiety. For the anxiety states that still mentioned neuroses in *DSM-III*, see 225–39.

132. John Feighner, "Nosology: A Voice for a Systematic Data-Oriented Approach," *American Journal of Psychiatry* 136 (1979): 1173–74, quote from 1173.

133. On the growing technical aspects of American medicine in general, see Adele E. Clarke et al., "Biomedicalization: Technoscientific Transformations of Health, Illness, and U.S. Biomedicine," *American Sociological Review* 68 (2003): 161–94.

134. Paul Chodoff, "*DSM-III* and Psychotherapy," *American Journal of Psychiatry* 143 (1986): 201–3, quote from 201.

135. Stephen Jay Gould pointed out that science, as an activity performed by humans, is constructed by human assumptions. See Stephen Jay Gould, *The Mismeasure of Man*, rev. ed. (New York: W. W. Norton, 1996).

136. Ethicist Carl Elliott has recently pointed out that clinical trials often attract a subculture of patients who have their own motives for participation. Carl Elliott, "Guinea-Pigging," *New Yorker*, January 7, 2008, 36–41.

137. One of the current screening instruments involves only two questions. See Simon Gilbody, David Richards, Stephen Brealey, and Catherine Hewitt, "Screening for Depression in Medical Settings with the Patient Health Questionnaire (PHQ): A Diagnostic Meta-Analysis," *Journal of General Internal Medicine* 22 (2007): 1596–1602.

138. For a description of some of the plans for the next edition of *DSM*, see Darrel A. Regier, William E. Narrow, Michael B. First, and Tina Marshall, "The APA Classification of Mental Disorders: Future Perspectives," *Psychopathology* 35 (2002): 166–70.

139. David Faust and Richard A. Miner, "The Empiricist and His New Clothes: *DSM-III* in Perspective," *American Journal of Psychiatry* 143 (1986): 962–67.

140. For more of an exploration of this issue, see Horwitz and Wakefield, *Loss of Sadness*.

141. For example, although the Church of Scientology is a relatively fringe movement, it has been extremely active in criticizing psychiatry and has organized widespread attacks on the profession through its offshoot group, the Citizens Commission on Human Rights. See, for example, Jan Eastgate, "The Case against Electroshock Treatment," *USA Today (Magazine)*, November 1998, 28–30. Kramer pointed out that the Scientologists helped to encourage popular hysteria about Prozac. Peter D. Kramer, *Listening to Prozac* (New York: Penguin Books, 1993), xviii.

Chapter 3 — American Moods and the Consumer Solution

1. "Pill to Fight Mental Depression," *Business Week*, April 13, 1963, 76–77.

2. Tone, "Listening to the Past"; Jonathan M. Metzl, "'Mother's Little Helper': The Crisis of Psychoanalysis and the Miltown Resolution," *Gender & History* 15 (2003): 228–55.

3. Jean M. Grow, Jin Seong Park, and Xiaoqi Han, "'Your Life is Waiting!': Symbolic Meanings in Direct-to-Consumer Antidepressant Advertising," *Journal of Communication Inquiry* 30 (2006): 163–88.

4. See Carl Elliott, *Better Than Well: American Medicine Meets the American Dream* (New York: W. W. Norton, 2003).

5. For this chapter, I analyzed 306 articles in popular magazines published between 1954 and 1990. These comprise most of the articles found by searching the *Reader's*

Guide to Popular Literature during these decades. I excluded periodicals that were directed more to a professional audience (such as *Science*) or those that merely reported on physician or scientific activities (such as *Science News*).

6. Kramer, *Listening to Prozac*.

7. E. B. White, "Yule Neurosis Sifted in Report," *New Yorker*, December 25, 1954, 19.

8. I am qualitatively separating periodicals based on content and target audience. For women's magazines, I include such standards as *Vogue, Ladies' Home Journal*, and *Good Housekeeping*. Health magazines include *Psychology Today* and *Prevention*. News magazines include *Time* and *Newsweek*, while general interest periodicals include *Reader's Digest* and *Saturday Evening Post*. For the concept of tracking differences in periodical type, I am indebted to Mark Micale, who suggested that I look at the 1958 classic work by Ellegard on popular magazine reception. Alvar Ellegard, *Darwin and the General Reader: The Reception of Darwin's Theory of Evolution in the British Periodical Press, 1859–1872* (Chicago: University of Chicago Press, 1990), republished from the 1958 edition.

9. Historians have pointed out that publishers tailored the content of their magazines based on consumer interest, particularly as reflected in sales. For a discussion of this a few decades earlier, see Douglas B. Ward, "The Reader as Consumer: Curtis Publishing Company and Its Audience, 1910–1930," *Journalism History* 22 (1996): 46–55.

10. See, for example, Gerald L. Klerman, "The Age of Youthful Melancholia: Depression and the Baby Boomers," *USA Today (Magazine)*, July 1988, 69–71; Gerald L. Klerman, "Age and Clinical Depression: Today's Youth in the Twenty-first Century," *Journal of Gerontology* 31 (1976): 318–23.

11. My approach toward the growth of consumer culture and depression's place within it is indebted to Lizbeth Cohen's exciting synthesis of the enormous expansion of consumer culture in post–World War II America. Lizbeth Cohen, *A Consumers' Republic: The Politics of Mass Consumption in Postwar America* (New York: Alfred A. Knopf, 2003).

12. There were thirty articles on anxiety and only nine on depression between 1951 and 1960. *Reader's Guide to Periodical Literature*.

13. There were 784 listings under "depression" in the Vanderbilt Television News Archive (http://tvnews.vanderbilt.edu) from 1968 to August 18, 2008. It was not until the early 1990s that "depression" was more often used to describe a mental state rather than an economic condition.

14. For the widespread popular influence of Freudian psychoanalysis, see Hale, *Rise and Crisis of Psychoanalysis*. For more on the general rise in acceptance of a psychological outlook in American society, see Herman, *Romance of American Psychology*; Eva S. Moskowitz, *In Therapy We Trust: America's Obsession with Self Fulfillment* (Baltimore: Johns Hopkins University Press, 2001).

15. See, for example, Karl Huber, "The Blues, and How to Chase Them," *McCall's*, August 1960, 98; David Elkind and J. Herbert Hamsher, "The Anatomy of Melancholy," *Saturday Review*, September 30, 1972, 54–59; Theodore Isaac Rubin, "Psychiatrist's Notebook," *Ladies' Home Journal*, May 1976, 26; Willard Gaylin, "Caring Makes the Difference," *Psychology Today*, August 1976, 34–39.

16. See, for example, Alice Kosner, "What to Do When You're *Really* Depressed," *McCall's*, November 1977, 221, 281–86; "Depression: When the Blues Become Serious," *Changing Times*, March 1978, 37–39.

17. "What You Should Know About Mental Depression: Interview with Dr. Bertram S.

Brown, Director, National Institute of Mental Health," *U.S. News & World Report*, September 9, 1974, 37–40, quote from 40. See chapter 5 for more details on Eagleton's case.

18. See, for example, Nathan S. Kline, *From Sad to Glad: Kline on Depression* (New York: Putnam, 1974). For more recent volumes, see, for example, Donald F. Klein and Paul H. Wender, *Understanding Depression: A Complete Guide to Its Diagnosis and Treatment* (New York: Oxford University Press, 2005); Dennis S. Charney and Charles B. Nemeroff, *The Peace of Mind Prescription: An Authoritative Guide to Finding the Most Effective Treatment for Anxiety and Depression* (New York: Houghton Mifflin, 2004). While these authors are better known in the psychiatric literature, their volumes have not sold as well as those written by popular writers or psychiatrists with less of a research background.

19. "The New Depression Treatments," *Harper's Bazaar*, September 1973, 159, 168. Brown also received national attention for his role in attempting to help courts and Congress make sense of growing criticism of lobotomy for psychiatric conditions. See, for example, Saul Friedman, "Senators Probe Brain Control Experiments," *Miami Herald*, February 24, 1973. (Thanks to Jeffrey Bernstein for calling my attention to Brown's national roles and for the newspaper citation.)

20. For an account of Knauth's experiences that emphasizes treatment, see Peter Stoler, "A Season in Hell," *Time*, March 31, 1975, 78–80.

21. Percy Knauth, "A Season in Hell," *Life*, June 9, 1972, 74–84, quote from 84. See also S. J. Anderson, "The Dark Void of Depression," *USA Today (Magazine)*, November 1988, 70–72.

22. Linda Marx, "'I Was Full of Terror and Fright,'" *People*, January 12, 1987, 35–36; Louis J. Slovinsky, "Out of Depression," *New York Times Magazine*, January 3, 1988, 36; Mary Kay Blakely, "Memories of Frank," *Psychology Today*, October 1989, 48–52.

23. Mary-Ellen Banashek, "Depression: How to Kick It," *Mademoiselle*, January 1977, 85, 140–44.

24. Joan Mills, "Breakdown! A Journey through Stress," *Reader's Digest*, January 1982, 49–53; Ann Roth, Arlene Eisenberg, and Howard Eisenberg, "Something Was Happening to My Husband," *Good Housekeeping*, October 1982, 66–74.

25. Jay M. Weiss, Howard I. Glazer, and Larissa A. Pohorecky, "Neurotransmitters and Helplessness: A Chemical Bridge to Depression?" *Psychology Today*, December 1974, 58–62.

26. On the history of vitamins in America, see Rima D. Apple, *Vitamania: Vitamins in American Culture* (New Brunswick, N.J.: Rutgers University Press, 1996).

27. Lee Salk, "When Someone You Love Is Depressed," *McCall's*, November 1980, 72. For more on the evolution of the concept of chemical imbalance, see Christopher M. France, Paul H. Lysaker, and Ryan Robinson, "The 'Chemical Imbalance' Explanation for Depression: Origins, Lay Endorsement, and Clinical Implications," *Professional Psychology: Research and Practice* 38 (2007): 411–20.

28. Zelda Segal and Julius Segal, "Twelve Myths About the Blues," *Seventeen*, September 1981, 140–41, 156; Jeff Jarvis, "Caught in a Terrifying Spiral of Depression, Kristy McNichol Is Rescued by Big Brother Jimmy," *People*, May 9, 1983, 69–73.

29. "Depression and Divorce," *Saturday Evening Post*, January 1982, 123–24.

30. "Foods to Help You Cope with Moods," *Glamour*, May 1978, 268; June Roth, "The Anti-Depression Diet," *Harper's Bazaar*, July 1982, 45–46, 149–50; "Depressed May Have a B6 Deficiency," *Prevention*, March 1985, 10–11; Sheila Sobell Moramarco,

"Food Blues?" *Vogue*, June 1983, 246. Writers began to report on the use of tyrosine and tryptophan, readily available nutrients that were used as pharmaceutical agents (the current term is "nutraceuticals"), in 1984. See, for example, "Depression Lifted with Tyrosine," *Prevention*, December 1984, 18. Although popular writers usually stressed the value of sleep to prevent depression, *Newsweek* reported in 1971 on some sleep deprivation experiments to alleviate depression in West Germany. On sleep issues in depression, see "Rx for Depression?" *Newsweek*, August 30, 1971, 61; Carin Rubenstein, "Sadness Succors the Sleepless," *Psychology Today*, February 1982, 76.

31. Linda Trop, "Hot Weather Downer," *American Health*, July-August 1988, 54; Ned Miller, "Season of Our Discontent," *Health*, July 1988, 20.

32. Andrea Linne, "A Test for Depression," *Family Health*, May 1981, 10–11; L.L., "Melancholy Baby," *Health*, March 1982, 32–33; Margot Slade, "A Blood Test for Depression," *Psychology Today*, October 1979, 33; M.L.S., "New Ways to Spot and Treat Depression," *Good Housekeeping*, October 1983, 205. On the X-ray analogy, see Emily Freeman, "Depression: New Treatments for Our Number One Mental Health Problem," *Better Homes and Gardens*, April 1982, 23–24, 28. See also Mary C. Love, "A Skin Test for Depression," *Psychology Today*, December 1984, 13. For other specific tests for mental illness, see, for example, Phyllis Malanka, "Fated for Mania?" *Health*, March 1985, 16.

33. Jamie Talan, "Deceptive Depression," *Psychology Today*, July 1988, 17; Joanna Torrey, "Am I Blue?" *Harper's Bazaar*, August 1988, 159, 192; Chris Raymond, "Good News About Menopause," *American Health*, November 1988, 52; Pamela King, "The (Meno)pause That Refreshes," *Psychology Today*, December 1988, 11.

34. "Happy Hearts: Preventing the Blues May Prevent Heart Attacks," *Prevention*, February 1989, 10–12.

35. See, for example, Laura Jack, "Is Your Body Bringing You Down?" *Mademoiselle*, September 1989, 154.

36. For information on the depression of famous figures in history, see, for example, Anne H. Rosenfeld, "Depression: Dispelling Despair," *Psychology Today*, June 1985, 28–34; Anthony Storr, "Winston Churchill's Black Dog," *Esquire*, January 1969, 95–99, 134–42; "Hunting 'The Black Dog,'" *U.S. News & World Report*, March 9, 1987, 102; Gregory Jaynes, "The Black Dog Blues," *Life*, December 1989, 24.

37. See, for example, Gideon G. Panter, "The Post-Holiday and Post-Baby Blues," *Parents*, December 1978, 34.

38. Moskowitz, *In Therapy We Trust*.

39. Janet Graham, "To Beat the Blues," *Reader's Digest*, April 1967, 39–40, 44–46.

40. "How to Beat the Blues," *Better Homes and Gardens*, February 1970, 116–17, 122. See also Judith Viorst, "How to Feel Better When You're Feeling Rotten," *Redbook*, May 1977, 68.

41. See, for example, "Vacation Blues," *USA Today (Magazine)*, April 1986, 13–14; Olivia Schleffelin Nordberg, "Post-Vacation Blues," *Parents*, September 1989, 112–14. On unhappiness with winter holidays, see, for example, Mark Rosin, "Christmas Depression and How to Deal with It," *Harper's Bazaar*, December 1972, 108–9, 122; Rita Goldman, "How to Cope with Holiday Hangups and Hangovers," *Harper's Bazaar*, December 1977, 134–35, 139.

42. Maxine Paetro, "How to Survive Happiness," *Mademoiselle*, October 1980, 219, 243–44; Susan Jacoby, "When 'Joyful' Occasions Get You Down," *McCall's*, November 1982, 32–37, 67; Mary Ellin Bruns, "The Sunday Blues," *Mademoiselle*,

March 1983, 252–53; Gail Kessler, "Why Getting What You Want Can Be a Downer," *Seventeen*, May 1986, 130–31; "Knock Those Sunday-Night Blues," *Glamour*, October 1986, 70.

43. "Exercise Plus: You and Feelings," *Vogue*, August 1980, 255, 284–85; Julia M. Klein, "Running Away from Depression," *Ms.*, May 1983, 85; Gail Kessler, "What to Do When You're Melancholy, Baby," *Mademoiselle*, March 1984, 48; Mary Numata, "Lifting Weights and Spirits," *Health*, December 1984, 18; Elizabeth Stark, "Exercising Away Depression," *Psychology Today*, December 1984, 68; William Gottlieb, "Headstrong: Exercise as Therapy," *Prevention*, July 1985, 61–63; Maggie Spilner, "Taking the High Road Out of Depression," *Prevention*, March 1989, 82–84; "Don't Just Sit There—Do Something," *Prevention*, May 1989, 10–11; Keith W. Johnsgard, "Peace of Mind," *Runner's World*, April 1990, 73–81. Some researchers noted in the late 1980s, however, that athletes were more prone to depression than their age-matched controls. Eleanor Grant, "Can Exercise Beat the Blues?" *Psychology Today*, September 1987, 22.

44. "How I Beat the Blues," *Good Housekeeping*, March 1976, 90–91; "What Stars Do to Shine," *Teen*, July 1986, 40.

45. Amitai Etzioni, "Christmas Blues," *Psychology Today*, December 1976, 23; Joann Ellison Rodgers, "Christmas Depression Syndrome," *Mademoiselle*, December 1977, 50; Marcia Lasswell and Norman Lobsenz, "Living Happily through the Holidays," *McCall's*, December 1977, 62–66, 172; Lewis Burke Frumkes, "Loneliness: Beating the Christmas Blues," *Harper's Bazaar*, December 1981, 86, 90; Bradley Hitchings, "How to Shake Those Holiday Blues," *Business Week*, December 10, 1984, 156–60; Robert Coles, "Dealing with the Holiday Blues," *New Choices for the Best Years*, December 1989, 74–75.

46. See, for example, "Good Listening: Music to Soothe, Calm, Lift the Holiday Blues," *Glamour*, December 1982, 40; "Away for the Holidays?" *USA Today (Magazine)*, December 1985, 14–15.

47. Barbara Hollan, "Depression Is the Pits, But You Don't Need Pills to Climb Out," *McCall's*, March 1983, 30–32, 147, quote from 30.

48. Hollan, "Depression Is the Pits," 147.

49. Joan R. Heilman, "Six Self-Help Tips to Rout the Blues," *Reader's Digest*, December 1983, 93–96.

50. "Dr. Kline Writes About Depression for Putnam," *Publishers Weekly*, May 6, 1974, 48; Nathan S. Kline, "Antidepressants May Bring New Life to Your Life," *Vogue*, July 1975, 104–5; Kline, *From Sad to Glad*. See also Cathy Perlmutter, "Beyond Thought Therapy," *Prevention*, October 1990, 50–52.

51. James A. Steck, "Drugs for Depression's Sadness," *Psychology Today*, July 1975, 16–17; Linda Wolfe, "When the Blues Don't Go Away," *McCall's*, 94–95, 132–35.

52. Wolfe, "When the Blues Don't Go Away."

53. Electroconvulsive therapy (ECT) was also mentioned as a possible treatment, usually in terms of how useful it could be despite its fearsome reputation. Maggie Scarf, "Shocking the Depressed Back to Life," *New York Times Magazine*, June 17, 1979, 32–34+; Harold A. Sackheim, "The Case for ECT," *Psychology Today*, June 1985, 36–40; Susan Squire, "Shock Therapy's Return to Respectability," *New York Times Magazine*, November 22, 1987, 78–79, 85–89. See also Laura D. Hirshbein and Sharmalie Sarvananda, "History, Power, and Electricity: American Popular Magazine Accounts of Electroconvulsive Therapy, 1940–2005," *Journal of the History of the Behavioral Sciences* 44 (2008): 1–18.

54. For historical analysis of consumer identity through use of medications, see Robert Bud, "Germophobia to the Care Free Life," in *Medicating Modern America: Prescription Drugs in History*, ed. Andrea Tone and Elizabeth Siegel Watkins (New York: New York University Press, 2007), 17–41.

55. Aaron Beck and Maria Kovacs, "A New, Fast Therapy for Depression," *Psychology Today*, January 1977, 94–102.

56. Marnie Severson, "Depression Discussion," *Health*, July 1982, 19–20.

57. Edward Ziegler, "*Think* Your Way Out of Depression," *Reader's Digest*, December 1980, 124–27; David D. Burns, *Feeling Good: The New Mood Therapy* (New York: Morrow, 1980). See also Valerie Adler, "'Accentuate the Positive': Thinking Happy Thoughts Sounds Corny but Beats the Blues," *American Health*, May 1989, 50.

58. Rosenfeld, "Depression"; Christopher Norwood, "The Great Depression: News About the Blues," *Mademoiselle*, May 1986, 186–87, 239–42; Carol Duchow Gurin, "Depression," *Ms.*, December 1987, 48–49, 52–54, 88.

59. John Leo, "Talk Is as Good as a Pill," *Time*, May 26, 1986, 60; Severson, "Depression Discussion."

60. As early as 1975, it was possible to have an extensive review of treatments available for depression that did not include any discussion of psychoanalysis. See, for example, "New Ways to Treat Depression," *Good Housekeeping*, July 1975, 149.

61. William Cole, "New Drugs for Depression," *Better Homes and Gardens*, April 1988, 66; Carolyn Jabs, "Depressed? This Will Cheer You Up," *McCall's*, November 1985, 84–87, 152.

62. Abigail Trafford, "New Hope for the Depressed," *U.S. News & World Report*, January 24, 1983, 39–42, quote from 39.

63. "Depression!" *Good Housekeeping*, March 1977, 28, 33, 36, 40–42; Heilman, "Six Self-Help Tips."

64. For the history of the upheavals in the 1960s, see Todd Gitlin, *The Sixties: Years of Hope, Days of Rage* (New York: Bantam Books, 1987). For a broad perspective on the 1970s, see Bruce J. Schulman, *The Seventies: The Great Shift in American Culture, Society, and Politics* (Cambridge: Da Capo Press, 2001).

65. "Coping with Depression," *Newsweek*, January 8, 1973, 51–54. See also Gerald M. Knox, "Blues Really Get You Down," *Better Homes and Gardens*, January 1974, 12–18.

66. "New Depression Treatments"; Cheryl Tevis, "Depression: Growing Occupational Hazard for Farmers," *Successful Farming*, January 1984, 30–31.

67. "New Ways to Treat Depression"; Marion Steinman, "Depression: Our Common Curse," *Saturday Evening Post*, December 1975, 54–55, 86. See also "Coping with Life's Strains," *U.S. News & World Report*, May 1, 1975, 80–82; "The Depression Epidemic," *USA Today (Magazine)*, April 1979, 15–16.

68. Marilyn Mercer, "The Complete Book of Depression," *Good Housekeeping*, October 1979, 91–96.

69. "Treating Depression," *Intellect*, March 1977, 299.

70. Aaron T. Beck and Jeffrey E. Young, "College Blues," *Psychology Today*, September 1978, 80–92. The estimates on college depression were significantly less alarming by the 1980s. A 1983 report stated that only 7 percent of college men had been seriously depressed the previous year. Phillip Shaver, "Down at College," *Psychology Today*, May 1983, 16.

71. Joyce Brothers, "Where to Turn for Help," *Good Housekeeping*, May 1971, 48, 50–53, quote from 50, ellipses in the original.

72. "Coping with Depression."

73. Alice Lake, "How to Cope—When You Feel You Can't," *Redbook*, January 1978, 81–85, 148, quote from 83.

74. Rona Cherry and Laurence Cherry, "The Common Cold of Mental Ailments: Depression," *New York Times Magazine*, November 25, 1973, 38, 117–27, 134–35.

75. Helen De Rosis and Victoria Y. Pellegrino, "Depression on the Job," *Harper's Bazaar*, January 1977, 57, 129, quote from 57.

76. Gerald L. Klerman, "The Age of Melancholy?" *Psychology Today*, April 1979, 37–42, 85. See also "It Isn't Easy Being Blue," *Current Health*, November 1979, 3–11; Knox, "Blues Really Get You Down."

77. "What Causes Mental Depression—and How to Cope," *U.S. News & World Report*, October 8, 1979, 39–40; Richard Grossman, "The Cash-Flow Syndrome," *Family Health*, June 1981, 8–9; Margot Slade, "Depressed? Try Friends," *Psychology Today*, October 1978, 19.

78. For a critique of 1980s optimism, see Harry Stein, "Rising Above Malaise," *Esquire*, February 1985, 35–36; Micheline Maynard, "Even Winners Battle the Blues," *U.S. News & World Report*, January 20, 1986, 55. For ways in which President Reagan's character affected popular culture, see Gil Troy, *Morning in America: How Ronald Reagan Invented the 1980s* (Princeton, N.J.: Princeton University Press, 2005).

79. T. Berry Brazelton, "The Withdrawn Child: Two Years," *Redbook*, November 1975, 76–82; "New Tools to Treat Mental Depression," *U.S. News & World Report*, May 25, 1981, 81; Lewis Burke Frumkes, "Is Your Youngster Depressed?" *Harper's Bazaar*, June 1983, 18–19, 155; "Dealing with Depression," *Current Health 2*, April 1985, 26–27. For news reports, see especially "Segment 3 (Depressed Children)," NBC Evening News, December 26, 1978; and "Illinois: Teenage Suicide," NBC Evening News, March 13, 1987, both in Vanderbilt Television News Archive.

80. Judi Marks, "What's Normal, What's Not?" *Teen*, February 1980, 9–10, 14, quote from 9.

81. "When a Teenager Gets Really Depressed," *Changing Times*, June 1982, 27–28.

82. See David Gelman et al., "Depression," *Newsweek*, May 4, 1987, 48–57. Gerald Klerman credited himself with coining the term "agent blue." Klerman, "Age of Youthful Melancholia."

83. "10 Ways to Beat the Blues," *Seventeen*, December 1978, 136–37, 148, quote from 136.

84. "Teenage Depression: Some Hope for Those Hopeless Feelings," *Teen*, September 1982, 6–8, 97–99; "Depressed? Here's Help for Hopeless Feelings," *Teen*, March 1985, 10, 14, 85.

85. Although the study of people in old age—gerontology—began in the years after World War II, the field picked up a great deal of momentum in the 1970s. See W. Andrew Achenbaum, *Crossing Frontiers: Gerontology Emerges as a Science* (New York: Cambridge University Press, 1995).

86. "Senility? It's More Likely Depression, Says Psychiatrist," *Retirement Living*, March 1977, 15. Depression could mask an underlying medical problem, too. Jonathan V. Wright, "A Case of Apathy and Depression," *Prevention*, June 1984, 113–18.

87. Larry W. Thompson and Dolores Gallagher, "Depression and Its Treatment in the Elderly," *Aging*, January 1985, 14–18, quote from 18. See also Alexandra Mezey, "Grandma Layton's Drawings Don't Just Reflect a Big Talent—They've Cured Her 40-Year Depression," *People*, February 24, 1986, 93–94; Louise Crooks, "Depression Can Be Conquered," *Modern Maturity*, October–November 1989, 10–11.

88. Helen Alpert, "10 Ways to Fight Depression," *Retirement Living*, June 1975, 31–33.

89. Storr, "Winston Churchill's Black Dog." See also Elkind and Hamsher, "Anatomy of Melancholy."

90. See, for example, "Melancholy and the Muse," *FDA Consumer*, October 1983, 18; John Leo, "The Ups and Downs of Creativity," *Time*, October 8, 1984, 76; Constance Holden, "Creativity and the Troubled Mind," *Psychology Today*, April 1987, 9–10; Judy Folkenberg, "Mad Artists?" *American Health*, June 1988, 85; "The Meticulous Melancholia of a Poet," *Discover*, May 1987, 12–13. The distinction between manic-depressive, or bipolar, disorder and major depression was not clearly made in the popular literature during this time period. Jamison and Andreasen generally reported on bipolar disorder, but the press reported the various kinds of mood disorders interchangeably. See, for example, Jeffrey Brune, "The Mad Genius Vindicated," *Health*, February 1987, 26. On bipolar disorder in American culture and society, see Emily Martin, *Bipolar Expeditions: Mania and Depression in American Culture* (Princeton, N.J.: Princeton University Press, 2007).

91. Alan S. Bellack, Michel Hersen, and Jonathan Himmelhoch, "Social Skills Training Compared with Pharmacotherapy and Psychotherapy in the Treatment of Unipolar Depression," *American Journal of Psychiatry* 138 (1981): 1562–67, quote from 1562.

92. "Treating Mood Disorders," *FDA Consumer*, July–August 1984, 4; Rosenfeld, "Depression."

93. Jane O'Hara, "The Depression Mystery," *World Press Review*, June 1984, 29–30.

94. Stoudemire et al., "Economic Burden of Depression."

95. Many of the major motion pictures of the 1970s were quite depressing or at least somewhat sad—even the comedies (for example, *Heaven Can Wait*). On the national pessimism as reflected in public policy, see David Brian Robertson, "Introduction: Loss of Confidence and Policy Change in the 1970s," *Journal of Policy History* 10 (1998): 1–18. Glen Gabbard has also pointed out that the 1970s were a time when psychiatrists (and physicians in general) were not well-respected authorities, so it is understandable that their interventions would not be more celebrated regarding depression. Glen O. Gabbard and Krin Gabbard, *Psychiatry and the Cinema*, 2nd ed. (Washington, D.C.: American Psychiatric Press, 1999), 133–46.

96. "What You Should Know About Mental Depression," 37. See also Susan Moskowitz, "How to Live with His Worst Moods," *Ladies' Home Journal*, February 1982, 55–62.

97. On efforts to understand "clinical" depression, see, for example, Ricki Lewis, "Down So Long It Looks Like Up?" *Health*, November 1983, 8; Claudia Wallis, "Is Mental Illness Inherited?" *Time*, March 9, 1987, 67; "Gene of the Week," *Time*, March 30, 1987, 62; Terence Monmaney, "When Manic Depression Is Part of the Family Legacy," *Newsweek*, May 4, 1987, 53; Harold Hopkins, "Calming the Roller Coaster of Mood Swings," *FDA Consumer*, November 1988, 21–25.

98. For the older literature on suicide, see, for example, Louis I. Dublin and Bessie Bunzel, *To Be, or Not to Be: A Study of Suicide* (New York: H. Smith and R. Haas, 1933); Emile Durkheim, *Suicide: A Study in Sociology*, trans. John A. Spaulding and George Simpson (Glencoe, Ill.: Free Press, 1951). For more on the history of suicide, see Howard I. Kushner, "American Psychiatry and the Cause of Suicide, 1844–1917," *Bulletin of the History of Medicine* 60 (1986): 36–57; Howard I. Kushner, *Self-Destruction in the Promised Land: A Psychocultural Biology of American Suicide*

(New Brunswick, N.J.: Rutgers University Press, 1989); Georges Minois, *History of Suicide: Voluntary Death in Western Culture*, trans. Lydia G. Cochrane (Baltimore: Johns Hopkins University Press, 1999).

99. Bryant H. Roisum, "How to Recognize Suicidal Depression," *Ladies' Home Journal*, September 1964, 26–28.

100. Arnold A. Hutschnecker, "If You're Depressed, Know Why," *Vogue*, January 15, 1972, 52–53, 101–3.

101. Jim Jerome, "Catching Them Before Suicide," *New York Times Magazine*, January 14, 1979, 30–33.

102. See also "Coping with Depression." Suicide prevention centers began to open in the 1960s in California and expanded throughout the country. See Louis I. Dublin, *Suicide: A Sociological and Statistical Study* (New York: Ronald Press, 1963).

103. "Coping with Life's Strains," 80.

104. See, for example, Sharon Carter, "Finding Help When You're Feeling Blue," *Vogue*, January 1986, 259.

105. Clive Wood, "Depressed About Life, or Just Depressed?" *Psychology Today*, February 1987, 22; Robert J. Trotter, "Stop Blaming Yourself," *Psychology Today*, February 1987, 31–39.

106. Carin Rubenstein, "Shunning the Depressed," *Psychology Today*, March 1982, 80–81; Anne H. Rosenfeld, "Coping with a Partner's Depression," *Psychology Today*, November 1987, 24; Holly Hall, "Weep and You Weep Alone," *Psychology Today*, June 1989, 18.

107. "A Man's Opinion: If Your Lover's in the Dumps, Help Him Out—But Don't Fall in Yourself," *Glamour*, April 1986, 124; Stephanie Renfrow Hamilton, "Are You Blue? How to Beat Depression," *Essence*, October 1986, 66–70, 130–34; Judith Stone, "Second-Hand Woes," *Glamour*, March 1987, 259.

108. Laurence Cherry, "The Good News About Depression," *New York*, June 2, 1986, 33–42, quote from 34.

109. See also Zelda Hedden-Sellman, "Cyclothymia: When Mood Swings Are Serious," *McCall's*, August 1987, 87; Winifred Gallagher, "Dysthymic Disorder: The DD's, Blues without End," *American Health*, April 1988, 80–88.

110. See, for example, Joan Costello, "Childhood Depression," *Parents*, December 1983, 117; Julius Segal and Zelda Segal, "Even Kids Get the 'Blues,'" *Parents*, November 1985, 208; David Elkind, "Depression," *Parents*, December 1987, 206; Lilian G. Katz, "More Than Just the Blues," *Parents*, June 1988, 190; James Comer, "Depressed Youngsters," *Parents*, October 1989, 237.

111. J.W.M., "Childhood Depression: The Hidden Disease," *Good Housekeeping*, April 1984, 300.

112. Sandra McCoy, "Danny's Descent into Hell," *Reader's Digest*, February 1986, 89–94.

113. Beverly McLeod, "Depressing News," *Psychology Today*, December 1984, 69; Eleanor Grant, "Depressed Moms: Mixed Messages for Kids," *Psychology Today*, October 1987, 14.

114. Kline, "Antidepressants May Bring New Life."

115. Clive Wood, "Sadder but Wiser," *Psychology Today*, January 1988, 8.

116. Lears described the origins of this process within the first few decades of the century. Lears, "From Salvation to Self-Realization."

117. Hazleton was also reported to have recognized that depression was a psychiatric concept, one not necessarily endorsed by psychologists. John Leo, "Learning to Live

with the Blues," *Time*, June 18, 1984, 91. See also Lesley Hazleton, "What's Good About Feeling Bad," *Vogue*, September 1984, 800–801; Lesley Hazleton, "Don't Feel Guilty About Sometimes Being Depressed," *Glamour*, October 1984, 123.

118. See, for example, Ami S. Brodoff, "Depression: Its Positive Side," *Vogue*, August 1984, 402.

119. Martin E. Seligman, "Boomer Blues," *Psychology Today*, October 1988, 50–55, quote from 55. For Seligman on learned helplessness, see, for example, Martin E. Seligman, J. Weiss, M. Weinraub, and A. Schulman, "Coping Behavior: Learned Helplessness, Physiological Change and Learned Inactivity," *Behaviour Research and Therapy* 18 (1980): 459–512.

120. Robert Hirschfeld, "Clinical Depression: When the Blues Won't Go Away," *McCall's*, March 1987, 88.

121. Dan Zevin, "Heartbreak Hotel," *Health*, January 1987, 18; "Post-Divorce Blues," *USA Today (Magazine)*, September 1989, 9.

122. See, for example, Wibo van de Linde, "His Strength Exhausted, Holland's Prince Claus Is Hospitalized for Severe Depression," *People*, November 1, 1982, 107.

123. Jarvis, "Caught in a Terrifying Spiral of Depression." One of the ways in which depression as explanation for celebrity problems manifested itself was as an explanation for substance abuse problems. See, for example, "Depression Almost Killed Ex-Manager Maury Wills," *Jet*, November 26, 1984, 46.

124. On the history of celebrity endorsements in advertisements in the early twentieth century, see Roland Marchand, *Advertising the American Dream: Making Way for Modernity, 1920–1940* (Berkeley: University of California Press, 1985); Jackson Lears, *Fables of Abundance: A Cultural History of Advertising in America* (New York: Basic Books, 1994).

125. Erica Goode, "Beating Depression," *U.S. News & World Report*, March 5, 1990, 48–56, quote from 48. See also Mary-Lane Kamberg, "A Sad State of Mind," *Current Health 2*, December 1989, 17–19; William Thomas Buckley, "You Can Beat Depression," *Reader's Digest*, February 1990, 173–76.

126. See Erica Goode, "Tailoring Treatment for Depression's Many Forms," *U.S. News & World Report*, March 5, 1990, 54–56.

127. Laura L. Smith and Charles H. Elliott, *Depression for Dummies* (New York: Wiley, 2003).

Chapter 4 — Gender, Depression, Diagnosis, and Power

1. H. A. Tomlinson, "The Puerperal Insanities," *American Journal of Insanity* 56 (1899): 69–88, quote from 70.

2. Yet as Regina Morantz-Sanchez has described, these kinds of arguments could be open to debate. Women physicians in the late nineteenth century objected to theories circulating at the time that women's reproductive cycles made them too debilitated for effort outside the home and engaged in studies that demonstrated this was not the case. See Regina Markell Morantz-Sanchez, *Sympathy and Science: Women Physicians in American Medicine* (New York: Oxford University Press, 1985), 53–56.

3. For the classic formulation of the differences between sex and gender, as well as the power of gender for historical analysis, see Joan W. Scott, "Gender: A Useful Category of Historical Analysis," *American Historical Review* 91 (1986): 1053–75.

4. A number of critics and historians have emphasized the coercive power of psychi-

atric institutions. See, in particular, Michel Foucault, *Madness and Civilization: A History of Insanity in the Age of Reason*, trans. R. Howard (New York: Pantheon, 1967); David J. Rothman, *The Discovery of the Asylum: Social Order and Disorder in the New Republic*, rev. ed. (Boston: Little, Brown, 1990); Andrew Scull, *Social Order/Mental Disorder: Anglo-American Psychiatry in Historical Perspective* (Berkeley: University of California Press, 1989). For more recent and nuanced views of the power negotiations within the asylum, see, for example, Roy Porter and David Wright, eds., *The Confinement of the Insane: International Perspectives, 1800–1965* (New York: Cambridge University Press, 2003).

5. For criticism about gender and diagnosis, see, for example, Paula J. Caplan and Lisa Cosgrove, eds., *Bias in Psychiatric Diagnosis* (Lanham, Md.: Jason Aronson, 2004).

6. Smith Ely Jelliffe, "Dispensary Work in Nervous and Mental Diseases," *Journal of Nervous and Mental Disease* 33 (1906): 234–41.

7. For historical context on gender, race, and class with regard to psychiatric diagnosis and neurasthenia in the early part of the century, see Francis G. Gosling and Joyce M. Ray, "The Right to Be Sick: American Physicians and Nervous Patients, 1885–1910," *Journal of Social History* 20 (1986): 251–67.

8. On nervous disorders in the American context, see Brad Campbell, "The Making of 'American': Race and Nation in Neurasthenic Discourse," *History of Psychiatry* 18 (2007): 157–78. On work and identity shifts for men in this time period, see E. Anthony Rotundo, *American Manhood: Transformations in Masculinity from the Revolution to the Modern Era* (New York: Basic Books, 1993); Olivier Zunz, *Making America Corporate, 1870–1920* (Chicago: University of Chicago Press, 1990); R. Marie Griffith, "Apostles of Abstinence: Fasting and Masculinity during the Progressive Era," *American Quarterly* 52 (2000): 599–638.

9. Warren L. Babcock, "On the Treatment of Acute and Curable Forms of Melancholia," *International Medical Magazine* 9 (1900): 1–6, quote from 1. Babcock was an assistant physician at the St. Lawrence State Hospital, Ogdensberg, New York.

10. Smith Ely Jelliffe, "Some Notes on Dispensary Work in Nervous and Mental Diseases," *Journal of Nervous and Mental Disease* 31 (1904): 309–17; Smith Ely Jelliffe, "Dispensary Work in Nervous and Mental Diseases," *Journal of Nervous and Mental Disease* 34 (1907): 691–98.

11. For Progressive-era concerns with efficiency, see Samuel Hays, *Conservation and the Gospel of Efficiency: The Progressive Conservation Movement, 1890–1920* (Cambridge, Mass.: Harvard University Press, 1959). Theodore Roosevelt was a key figure in the conservation movement, and Hays points out that Roosevelt made the connection between conservation and health. For Roosevelt and prevailing masculine ideals, see Neil Edward Stubbs, "Theodore Roosevelt and Ernest Hemingway: A Study in Two Strenuous Lives," *Theodore Roosevelt Association Journal* 25 (2002): 9–14; Gail Bederman, *Manliness and Civilization: A Cultural History of Gender and Race in the United States, 1880–1917* (Chicago: University of Chicago Press, 1995), 170–215.

12. For some of the gender differences in nervous disorders in the nineteenth century, see Kathleen Spies, "Figuring the Neurasthenic: Thomas Eakins, Nervous Illness, and Gender in Victorian America," *Nineteenth-Century Studies* 12 (1998): 84–109.

13. Mark Micale has pointed out that the demise of hysteria as a diagnosis paralleled the introduction of new diagnostic systems in Germany and the United States. Micale,

Approaching Hysteria, 169–75. Micale has recently described the little known history of hysteria in men in *Hysterical Men: The Hidden History of Male Nervous Disorder* (Cambridge, Mass.: Harvard University Press, 2008). For a classic analysis of nineteenth-century hysteria in women, see Carroll Smith-Rosenberg, "The Hysterical Woman: Sex Roles and Role Conflict in 19th-Century America," *Social Research* 39 (1972): 652–78. See also Elaine Showalter, *Hystories: Hysterical Epidemics and Modern Media* (New York: Columbia University Press, 1997), 30–61.

14. Ernest Jones, "The Treatment of the Neuroses, Including the Psychoneuroses," in *The Modern Treatment of Nervous and Mental Diseases*, ed. William A. White and Smith Ely Jelliffe (Philadelphia: Lea & Febiger, 1913), 331–416, quote from 357.

15. Francis X. Dercum, "Group II—Melancholia, Mania, Circular Insanity (Melancholia-Mania; Manic-Depressive Insanity)," in *A Clinical Manual of Mental Diseases* (Philadelphia: W. B. Saunders, 1913), 62–105.

16. Horatio M. Pollock, "Mental Disease in the United States in Relation to Environment, Sex and Age, 1922," *American Journal of Psychiatry* 82 (1925): 219–32.

17. Horatio M. Pollock, "Recurrence of Attacks in Manic-Depressive Psychoses," *American Journal of Psychiatry* 88 (1931): 567–74.

18. Roger S. Cohen, "The Mild Depressive Reactions," *Medical Annals of the District of Columbia* 3 (1934): 162–69.

19. See, for example, Hills, "Statistical Study of One Thousand Patients."

20. See, for example, A. J. Rosanoff, "Exciting Causes in Psychiatry," *American Journal of Insanity* 69 (1912): 351–401; E. E. Southard and Earl D. Bond, "Clinical and Anatomical Analysis of 25 Cases of Mental Disease Arising in the Fifth Decade, with Remarks on the Melancholia Question and Further Observations on the Distribution of Cortical Pigments," *American Journal of Insanity* 70 (1914): 779–828; Joseph C. Yaskin, "The Feeling of Unreality as a Differential Symptom of Mild Depressions," *Archives of Neurology and Psychiatry* 33 (1935): 368–78; Hohman, "Review of One Hundred and Forty-four Cases."

21. See, for example, Charles E. Gibbs, "Sexual Behavior and Secondary Sexual Hair in Female Patients with Manic-Depressive Psychoses, and the Relation of These Factors to Dementia Praecox," *American Journal of Psychiatry* 81 (1924): 41–56. For the medical construction of sexual deviation and mental disorder, see Henry L. Minton, "Femininity in Men and Masculinity in Women: American Psychiatry and Psychology Portray Homosexuality in the 1930s," *Journal of Homosexuality* 13 (1986): 1–22.

22. For an important exploration of gender, mental health, and illness in this time period, see Lunbeck, *Psychiatric Persuasion*.

23. Abraham Myerson conducted a survey in the late 1930s of psychiatrists, neurologists, and psychologists to see how these professionals felt about psychoanalysis. He found that while a large number of them were sympathetic to some of Freud's ideas, there were relatively few in any of the specialty groups who were entirely sold on Freud's system of psychoanalysis. Myerson, "Attitude of Neurologists, Psychiatrists and Psychologists."

24. For Kraepelin's description, see Emil Kraepelin, *Clinical Psychiatry* (New York: Macmillan, 1907).

25. See, for example, Monica Helen Green, *Women's Healthcare in the Medieval West: Texts and Contexts* (Aldershot: Ashgate, 2000); Mary E. Fissell, *Vernacular Bodies: The Politics of Reproduction in Early Modern England* (New York: Oxford University Press, 2004).

26. For an exploration of the issues that nineteenth-century British psychiatrists projected onto their women patients who appeared insane in the context of childbirth, see Hilary Marland, "Disappointment and Desolation: Women, Doctors and Interpretations of Puerperal Insanity in the Nineteenth Century," *History of Psychiatry* 14 (2003): 303–20.

27. George Stockton, "Melancholia and Its Treatment," *Philadelphia Medical Journal* 8 (1901): 571–73, quote from 571.

28. Henry M. Swift, "The Prognosis of Recurrent Insanity of the Manic Depressive Type," *American Journal of Insanity* 64 (1907): 311–26.

29. See G. M. Davidson, "Concerning Schizophrenia and Manic-Depressive Psychosis Associated with Pregnancy and Childbirth," *American Journal of Psychiatry* 92 (1936): 1331–46; William A. Horwitz and Meyer M. Harris, "Study of a Case of Cyclic Psychic Disturbances Associated with Menstruation," *American Journal of Psychiatry* 92 (1936): 1403–12.

30. For the history of gynecology, see Deborah Kuhn McGregor, *From Midwives to Medicine: The Birth of American Gynecology* (New Brunswick, N.J.: Rutgers University Press, 1998).

31. William A. White, "The Geographical Distribution of Insanity in the United States," *Journal of Nervous and Mental Disease* 30 (1903): 257–79, quote from 262. For a fascinating account of the intersection of gender and surgery in late-nineteenth-century gynecology, see Regina Morantz-Sanchez, *Conduct Unbecoming a Woman: Medicine on Trial in Turn-of-the-Century Brooklyn* (New York: Oxford University Press, 1999).

32. E. Ballentine, "A Study of the Outcome of Agitated Depressions of the Involution Period in Women," *State Hospital Bulletin* 5 (1912): 47–62, quote from 47–48.

33. Gerald Grob has pointed out that the average age of those in mental institutions had begun to climb by the end of the nineteenth century as the hospitals began to take on the function of what were in effect nursing homes (before such homes were built). See Grob, *Mental Illness and American Society*, 180–87.

34. Mary F. Brew, "A Study of Precipitating Factors in Involution Melancholia," *State Hospital Quarterly* 10 (1925): 422–28, quote from 428.

35. Gerald H. J. Pearson, "An Interpretative Study of Involutional Depression," *American Journal of Psychiatry* 85 (1928): 289–335.

36. Eleanora B. Saunders, "A Study of Depressions in Late Life with Special Reference to Content," *American Journal of Psychiatry* 88 (1932): 925–54, quote from 925. Saunders graduated from the Medical College of South Carolina and caused some friction in one of her early professional positions (at the South Carolina State Hospital) by insisting on scientific method (including laboratory studies). At the time when she wrote on involutional melancholia, Saunders was at the Sheppard Pratt Hospital in Baltimore. Peter McCandless, *Moonlight, Magnolias, and Madness: Insanity in South Carolina from the Colonial Period to the Progressive Era* (Chapel Hill: University of North Carolina Press, 1996), 308–13; Uta Anderson, "Eleanora Bennette Saunders: A Pioneering Psychiatrist," *Journal of the South Carolina Medical Association* 93 (1997): 223–26.

37. Wm. Malamud, S. L. Sands, and I. Malamud, "The Involutional Psychoses: A Socio-Psychiatric Study," *Psychosomatic Medicine* 3 (1941): 410–26. The concept of adjustment had widespread use in the early twentieth century, and many borrowed the language originally used to describe child guidance in order to discuss adjustment to old age. Psychologists G. Stanley Hall and Lillien Martin expanded work

they had done on children and adjustment for older people and their adjustment. G. Stanley Hall, *Senescence: The Last Half of Life* (New York: Appleton, 1922); Lillien J. Martin and Clare De Gruchy, *Salvaging Old Age* (New York: Macmillan, 1930).

38. See, for example, E. V. Eyman et al., "A Statistical Survey of the Biogenesis of Involutional Melancholia," *Diseases of the Nervous System* 3 (1942): 16–20.

39. For the emergence of psychology within the general field of social sciences in the late nineteenth and early twentieth centuries, see Dorothy Ross, *The Origins of American Social Science* (New York: Cambridge University Press, 1991); Thomas L. Haskell, *The Emergence of Professional Social Science: The American Social Science Association and the Nineteenth-Century Crisis of Authority* (Baltimore: Johns Hopkins University Press, 1977). For the role of testing in psychology, see Michael M. Sokal, ed., *Psychological Testing and American Society, 1890–1930* (New Brunswick, N.J.: Rutgers University Press, 1987).

40. Lewis M. Terman and Catharine Cox Miles, *Sex and Personality: Studies in Masculinity and Femininity* (New York: Russell & Russell, 1936); Henry L. Minton, "Community Empowerment and the Medicalization of Homosexuality: Constructing Sexual Identities in the 1930s," *Journal of the History of Sexuality* 6 (1996): 435–58.

41. Beulah Bosselman and Bernard Skorodin, "Masculinity and Femininity in Psychotic Patients: As Measured by the Terman-Miles Interest-Attitude Analysis Test," *American Journal of Psychiatry* 97 (1940): 699–702, quote from 700.

42. See, for example, G. H. Stevenson and S. R. Montgomery, "Paranoid Reaction Occurring in Women of Middle Age," *American Journal of Psychiatry* 88 (1932): 911–23; Harold D. Palmer, Donald W. Hastings, and Stephen H. Sherman, "Therapy in Involutional Melancholia," *American Journal of Psychiatry* 97 (1941): 1086–1115.

43. For psychoanalytic emphasis on the mother's role with children, see Janet Sayers, *Mothers of Psychoanalysis: Helene Deutsch, Karen Horney, Anna Freud, and Melanie Klein* (New York: W. W. Norton, 1993).

44. Cowles, "Progress in the Clinical Study of Psychiatry"; White, "Types in Mental Disease"; Abbot, "Forms of Insanity." The British clinician George Louis Dreyfus in the late nineteenth century apparently disagreed that involutional melancholia had a different prognosis, and persuaded Emil Kraepelin to take it out of his influential nosology. Farrar, "On the Methods of Later Psychiatry." See also Jackson, *Melancholia and Depression*, 207–11. For an argument that menopause was not the cause of psychosis (and that involutional melancholia therefore did not exist), see J. W. Courtney, "Concerning the Raison D'Etre of the Term 'Involutional' as Applied to Melancholia," *Boston Medical and Surgical Journal* 174 (1916): 416–18.

45. August Hoch and John T. MacCurdy, "The Prognosis of Involution Melancholia," *American Journal of Psychiatry* 78 (1922): 433–73. Hoch was deceased at the time of this publication.

46. Frank Fenwick Young, "Involution Melancholia," *New Orleans Medical & Surgical Journal* 83 (1930): 375–79.

47. For historical discussion of menopause, see Judith A. Houck, *Hot and Bothered: Women, Medicine, and Menopause in Modern America* (Cambridge, Mass.: Harvard University Press, 2006); Lois W. Banner, *In Full Flower: Aging Women, Power, and Sexuality* (New York: Vintage Books, 1992); S. E. Bell, "Changing Ideas: The Medicalization of Menopause," in *The Meanings of Menopause: Historical, Medical, and Clinical Perspectives*, ed. R. Formanek (Hillsdale, N.J.: Analytic Press, 1990), 43–63.

48. See, for example, Maurice Grozin, "Involution Melancholia," *Medical Review of Reviews* 37 (1931): 397–402; G. R. Jameison and James H. Wall, "Mental Reactions at the Climacterium," *American Journal of Psychiatry* 88 (1932): 895–909; Harold D. Palmer and Stephen H. Sherman, "The Involutional Melancholia Process," *Archives of Neurology and Psychiatry* 40 (1938): 762–88.

49. See, for example, Edward A. Strecker and Baldwin L. Keyes, "Ovarian Therapy in Involutional Melancholia," *New York Medical Journal* 116 (1922): 30–34; Karl M. Bowman and Lauretta Bender, "The Treatment of Involution Melancholia with Ovarian Hormone," *American Journal of Psychiatry* 88 (1932): 867–93. For the history of hormone preparations in the early twentieth century, see Diana Long Hall, "Biology, Sex Hormones and Sexism in the 1920's," *Philosophical Forum* 5 (1973–74): 81–96.

50. C. B. Farrar and Ruth MacLachlan Franks, "Menopause and Psychosis," *American Journal of Psychiatry* 87 (1931): 1031–44.

51. Eugene Davidoff, E. C. Reifenstein, and Gerald L. Goodstone, "The Treatment of Involutional Psychoses with Diethyl Stilbestrol," *American Journal of Psychiatry* 99 (1943): 557–64.

52. August A. Werner, Louis H. Kohler, C. C. Ault, and Emmett F. Hoctor, "Involutional Melancholia: Probable Etiology and Treatment," *Archives of Neurology and Psychiatry* 35 (1936): 1076–80.

53. C. C. Ault, Louis H. Hoctor, and August A. Werner, "Involutional Melancholia: Additional Report," *American Journal of Psychiatry* 97 (1940): 691–94, quote from 691.

54. C. C. Ault, Louis H. Hoctor, and August A. Werner, "Theelin Therapy in the Psychoses," *Journal of the American Medical Association* 109 (1937): 1786–88. See also August A. Werner, Louis H. Hoctor, and C. C. Ault, "Involutional Melancholia: A Review with Additional Cases," *Archives of Neurology and Psychiatry* 45 (1941): 944–52.

55. For the broader history of hormone therapy, see Elizabeth Siegel Watkins, *The Estrogen Elixir: A History of Hormone Replacement Therapy in America* (Baltimore: Johns Hopkins University Press, 2007).

56. Purcell G. Schube, M. C. McManamy, C. E. Trapp, and G. F. Houser, "Involutional Melancholia: Treatment with Theelin," *Archives of Neurology and Psychiatry* 38 (1937): 505–12.

57. Herbert S. Ripley, Ephraim Shorr, and George N. Papanicolaou, "The Effect of Treatment of Depression in the Menopause with Estrogenic Hormone," *American Journal of Psychiatry* 96 (1940): 905–13.

58. A. E. Bennett and C. B. Wilbur, "Convulsive Shock Therapy in Involutional States after Complete Failure with Previous Estrogenic Treatment," *American Journal of the Medical Sciences* 208 (1944): 170–76; Eugene Davidoff and Angelo Raffaele, "Electric Shock Therapy in Involutional Psychoses," *Journal of Nervous and Mental Disease* 99 (1944): 397–405.

59. See, for example, Lawrence Kurzrok, Charles H. Birnberg, and Seymour Livingston, "The Treatment of Female Menopause with Male Sex Hormone," *Endocrinology* 24 (1939): 347–50.

60. Herbert S. Ripley and George N. Papanicolaou, "The Menstrual Cycle with Vaginal Smear Studies in Schizophrenia, Depression and Elation," *American Journal of Psychiatry* 98 (1942): 567–73, quote from 567.

61. For the history of the Pap smear, see Monica J. Casper and Adele E. Clarke, "Making

the Pap Smear into the 'Right Tool' for the Job: Cervical Cancer Screening in the USA, circa 1940–1995," *Social Studies of Science* 28 (1998): 255–90.

62. Isadore Leo Fishbein, "Involutional Melancholia and Convulsive Therapy," *American Journal of Psychiatry* 106 (1949): 128–35.

63. Bureau of the Census, *Statistical Abstract of the United States, 1942* (Washington, D.C.: U.S. Government Printing Office, 1943), 95–96. The 1950 report indicated an even higher percentage of men within the total institutionalized patient population (65 percent men and 34 percent women). Bureau of the Census, *Statistical Abstract of the United States, 1950* (Washington, D.C.: U.S. Government Printing Office, 1950), 30. It is certainly possible that some of the differences in the literature regarding sex distribution of patients was due to differences between public and private psychiatric hospitals.

64. For some of the rich and complex history around medical approaches toward venereal disease, including syphilis, see Elizabeth Fee, "Sin vs. Science: Venereal Disease in Baltimore in the Twentieth Century," *Journal of the History of Medicine and Allied Sciences* 43 (1988): 141–64; Allan M. Brandt, *No Magic Bullet: A Social History of Venereal Disease in the United States since 1880* (New York: Oxford University Press, 1987).

65. Paul E. Huston and Lillian M. Locher, "Manic-Depressive Psychosis: Course When Treated and Untreated with Electric Shock," *Archives of Neurology and Psychiatry* 60 (1948): 37–48.

66. See, for example, Eugene Ziskind, Esther Somerfeld-Ziskind, and Louis Ziskind, "Metrazol Therapy in the Affective Psychoses," *Journal of Nervous and Mental Disease* 95 (1942): 460–73; Eugene Ziskind, Esther Somerfeld-Ziskind, and Louis Ziskind, "Metrazol and Electric Convulsive Therapy of the Affective Psychoses," *Archives of Neurology and Psychiatry* 53 (1945): 212–17; Benjamin Malzberg, "The Outcome of Electric Shock Therapy in the New York Civil State Hospitals," *Psychiatric Quarterly* 17 (1943): 154–63; Leon Reznikoff, "Indications and Results of Electric Shock Therapy in Mental Disorders," *Psychiatric Quarterly* 17 (1943): 355–63; Paul E. Huston and Lillian M. Locher, "Involutional Psychosis: Course When Untreated and When Treated with Electric Shock," *Archives of Neurology and Psychiatry* 59 (1948): 385–94.

67. Joel Braslow and Jack Pressman have addressed these possibilities in their work. Braslow, *Mental Ills and Bodily Cures*; Pressman, *Last Resort*. Braslow and Starks have also suggested that physicians were reluctant to use lobotomy with men because it would make them childlike and dependent. Joel T. Braslow and Sarah Linsley Starks, "The Making of Contemporary American Psychiatry, Part 2: Therapeutics and Gender before and after World War II," *History of Psychology* 8 (2005): 271–88.

68. The most recent history of the most common form of shock therapy, electroconvulsive therapy (ECT), does not mention this issue at all. Shorter and Healy, *Shock Therapy*.

69. See Denber and Bird, "Chlorpromazine in the Treatment of Mental Illness," 1021; Barsa and Kline, "Depression Treated with Chlorpromazine and Promethazine"; Ferreira and Freeman, "Clinical Trial of Marsilid"; Wilson G. Scanlon and William M. White, "Iproniazid (Marsilid): Its Use in Office Treatment of Depression," *American Journal of Psychiatry* 114 (1958): 1036–37; Azima and Vispo, "Imipramine"; Pollock, "Clinical Findings in the Use of Tofranil."

70. See, for example, Turner, O'Neill, and Merlis, "Treatment of Depression in Hospital-

ized Patients"; Donald F. Klein and Max Fink, "Psychiatric Reaction Patterns to Imipramine," *American Journal of Psychiatry* 119 (1962): 432–38; Saul H. Rosenthal, "Changes in a Population of Hospitalized Patients with Affective Disorders, 1945–1965," *American Journal of Psychiatry* 123 (1966): 671–81; Gerald L. Klerman and Eugene S. Paykel, "Depressive Pattern, Social Background, and Hospitalization," *Journal of Nervous and Mental Disease* 150 (1970): 466–78.

71. See note 63, this chapter.

72. Bureau of the Census, *Statistical Abstract of the United States, 1963* (Washington, D.C.: U.S. Government Printing Office, 1963), 86. Interestingly enough, there was a category in the 1960 census data identified as "without mental disorder"—yet these patients were clearly still in psychiatric hospitals (1,798 men and 707 women). If this number represented some kind of exercise of state authority, it clearly affected more men than women.

73. Joe Dorzab, Max Baker, Remi J. Cadoret, and George Winokur, "Depressive Disease: Familial Psychiatric Illness," *American Journal of Psychiatry* 127 (1971): 1128–33.

74. Fritz A. Freyhan, "The Modern Treatment of Depressive Disorders," *American Journal of Psychiatry* 116 (1960): 1057–64, quote from 1062.

75. See, for example, Alberto DiMascio et al., "Differential Symptom Reduction by Drugs and Psychotherapy in Acute Depression," *Archives of General Psychiatry* 36 (1979): 1450–56; Bruce J. Rounsaville, Brigitte A. Prusoff, and Nancy Padian, "The Course of Nonbipolar, Primary Major Depression: A Prospective 16-Month Study of Ambulatory Patients," *Journal of Nervous and Mental Disease* 168 (1980): 406–11.

76. See, for example, Myrna M. Weissman, Gerald L. Klerman, and Eugene S. Paykel, "Clinical Evaluation of Hostility in Depression," *American Journal of Psychiatry* 128 (1971): 261–66; Gerald L. Klerman et al., "Treatment of Depression by Drugs and Psychotherapy," *American Journal of Psychiatry* 131 (1974): 186–91; Weissman, Kasl, and Klerman, "Follow-Up of Depressed Women after Maintenance Treatment." Weissman and Klerman were not the only ones to study only women and then generalize to everyone. See also Eva Y. Deykin and Alberto DiMascio, "Relationship of Patient Background Characteristics to Efficacy of Pharmacotherapy in Depression," *Journal of Nervous and Mental Disease* 155 (1972): 209–15.

77. Myrna M. Weissman and Gerald L. Klerman, "The Chronic Depressive in the Community: Unrecognized and Poorly Treated," *Comprehensive Psychiatry* 18 (1977): 523–32. The book that encapsulated many of Weissman's findings did explain that the studies were performed on women. Myrna M. Weissman and Eugene S. Paykel, *The Depressed Woman: A Study of Social Relationships* (Chicago: University of Chicago Press, 1974).

78. See, for example, Brigitte A. Prusoff, Donald H. Williams, Myrna M. Weissman, and Boris M. Astrachan, "Treatment of Secondary Depression in Schizophrenia: A Double-Blind, Placebo-Controlled Trial of Amitriptyline Added to Perphenazine," *Archives of General Psychiatry* 36 (1979): 569–75.

79. Robert J. Bielski and Robert O. Friedel, "Prediction of Tricyclic Antidepressant Response: A Critical Review," *Archives of General Psychiatry* 33 (1976): 1479–89, quote from 1488.

80. One 1970 study had a total sample of seventy-four patients, only six of whom were men. The authors did not mention this as an issue. See Anthony LaPolla and Harry Jones, "Placebo-Control Evaluation of Desipramine in Depression," *American Journal of Psychiatry* 127 (1970): 335–38.

81. See, for example, John Feighner, "A Comparative Trial of Fluoxetine and Amitriptyline in Patients with Major Depressive Disorder," *Journal of Clinical Psychiatry* 46 (1985): 369–72; Karl Rickels et al., "Comparison of Two Dosage Regimens of Fluoxetine in Major Depression," *Journal of Clinical Psychiatry* 46 (1985): 38–41; Paul Stark and C. David Hardison, "A Review of Multicenter Controlled Studies of Fluoxetine vs. Imipramine and Placebo in Outpatients with Major Depressive Disorder," *Journal of Clinical Psychiatry* 46 (1985): 53–58.

82. Some estimate a prevalence of sexual side effects as high as 80 percent, but the data in this area is limited. R. C. Rosen, R. M. Lane, and M. Menza, "Effects of SSRIs on Sexual Function: A Critical Review," *Journal of Clinical Psychopharmacology* 19 (1999): 67–85.

83. A recent review on the subject of gender and depression by two well-respected researchers claimed that there was little information available about women's response to antidepressant medications because clinical trials in the past had not included women of childbearing years. Based on my review of the older clinical trials, this assertion is not true. Susan G. Kornstein and Diane M. E. Sloan, "Depression and Gender," in *The American Psychiatric Publishing Textbook of Mood Disorders*, ed. Dan J. Stein, David J. Kupfer, and Alan F. Schatzberg (Washington, D.C.: American Psychiatric Publishing, 2006), 687–98.

84. On the history of heart disease and hypertension research and its lack of applicability to women in the past, see Joan L. Thomas and Patricia A. Braus, "Coronary Artery Disease in Women: A Historical Perspective," *Archives of Internal Medicine* 158 (1998): 333–37; Teresa S. M. Tsang, Marion E. Barnes, Bernard J. Gersh, and Sharonne N. Hayes, "Risks of Coronary Heart Disease in Women: Current Understanding and Evolving Concepts," *Mayo Clinic Proceedings* 75 (2000): 1289–1303; Joseph Palca, "Women Left Out at NIH," *Science* 248 (1990): 1601–2; Ruth B. Merkatz et al., "Women in Clinical Trials of New Drugs," *New England Journal of Medicine* 329 (1993): 292–96.

85. For more on this, see chapter 2.

86. Although researchers occasionally acknowledged that estrogen is present in men—albeit at lower concentrations—they tended to discuss estrogen as though it were purely a female hormone.

87. Edward L. Klaiber et al., "Effects of Estrogen Therapy on Plasma MAO Activity and EEG Driving Responses of Depressed Women," *American Journal of Psychiatry* 128 (1972): 1492–98, quote from 1497.

88. Edward L. Klaiber, Donald M. Broverman, William Vogel, and Yutaka Kobayashi, "Estrogen Therapy for Severe Persistent Depressions in Women," *Archives of General Psychiatry* 36 (1979): 550–54. Klaiber remained attached to the idea that hormones affect women's emotional lives. See Edward L. Klaiber, *Hormones and the Mind* (New York: HarperCollins, 2001).

89. Ian C. Wilson, Arthur J. Prange, and Patricio Lara, "Methyltestosterone with Imipramine in Men: Conversion of Depression to Paranoid Reaction," *American Journal of Psychiatry* 131 (1974): 21–24, quotes from 21, 23. This paper did not mention that testosterone is found in small quantities in women, but rather assumed that testosterone was a hormone specific to men. Wilson and his group refer to imipramine's greater effectiveness in men, but I have not found other references that support this assertion.

90. Researchers continued to ask questions about the relationship of depression to menopause, even when they could find no relationship. See, for example, George

Winokur, "Depression in the Menopause," *American Journal of Psychiatry* 130 (1973): 92–93.

91. Dean Schuyler, *The Depressive Spectrum* (New York: Jason Aronson, 1974), 43.

92. For Menninger's public education efforts, see William C. Menninger, *Psychiatry in a Troubled World: Yesterday's War and Today's Challenge* (New York: Macmillan, 1948). For Menninger's expressions in relationship to the broader psychoanalytic movement, see Rebecca Jo Plant, "William Menninger and American Psychoanalysis, 1946–48," *History of Psychiatry* 16 (2005): 181–202. For the history of the Menninger family's influence, see Lawrence J. Friedman, *Menninger: The Family and the Clinic* (New York: Knopf, 1990).

93. Elaine Tyler May, *Homeward Bound: American Families in the Cold War Era* (New York: Basic Books, 1988). For more on masculinity in this time period, see K. A. Cuordileone, *Manhood and American Political Culture in the Cold War* (New York: Routledge, 2005).

94. One 1966 author described his experience with depressed and clingy women who were so demanding that the treatment team put them in groups out of desperation—to their surprise, the groups helped the women improve and helped them to be less dependent on their physicians. Paul R. Miller and Louise Ferone, "Group Psychotherapy with Depressed Women," *American Journal of Psychiatry* 123 (1966): 701–5.

95. James L. Evans, "Psychiatric Illness in the Physician's Wife," *American Journal of Psychiatry* 122 (1965): 159–63, quote from 162. For similar discussions of marital dynamics, see Robert L. DuPont Jr. and Henry Grunebaum, "Willing Victims: The Husbands of Paranoid Women," *American Journal of Psychiatry* 125 (1968): 151–59; Chester A. Pearlman, "Separation Reactions of Married Women," *American Journal of Psychiatry* 126 (1970): 946–50.

96. This pattern was evident in literature on women who were not psychiatric patients themselves but were the wives of men with alcoholism. One 1966 paper sharply criticized women's unresolved conflicts that led them to seek out men whom they could dominate—thus the women worsened their husbands' addictions by constantly trying to dominate them. These gender assumptions were not just held by male psychiatrists—two of the authors of the paper were women. Susan D. Taylor, Mary Wilbur, and Robert Osnos, "The Wives of Drug Addicts," *American Journal of Psychiatry* 123 (1966): 585–91.

97. For an excellent review of feminist opposition to psychiatry, see Nancy Tomes, "Feminist Histories of Psychiatry," in Micale and Porter, *Discovering the History of Psychiatry*, 348–83. For other groups' objections to psychiatry in the same time period, see Norman Dain, "Critics and Dissenters: Reflections on 'Anti-Psychiatry' in the United States," *Journal of the History of the Behavioral Sciences* 25 (1989): 3–25.

98. Betty Friedan, *The Feminine Mystique* (New York: Dell, 1963).

99. See, for example, Barbara Ehrenreich and Deirdre English, *For Her Own Good: 150 Years of the Experts' Advice to Women* (Garden City, N.Y.: Anchor Press, 1978); Phyllis Chesler, *Women and Madness* (New York: Avon Books, 1972); Elaine Showalter, *The Female Malady: Women, Madness, and English Culture, 1830–1980* (New York: Penguin Books, 1985).

100. See, for example, Anne M. Seiden, "Overview: Research on the Psychology of Women. I. Gender Differences and Sexual and Reproductive Life," *American Journal of Psychiatry* 133 (1976): 995–1007; Anne M. Seiden, "Overview: Research on the

Psychology of Women. II. Women in Families, Work, and Psychotherapy," *American Journal of Psychiatry* 133 (1976): 1111–23; Elaine (Hilberman) Carmen, Nancy Felipe Russo, and Jean Baker Miller, "Inequality and Women's Mental Health: An Overview," *American Journal of Psychiatry* 138 (1981): 1319–30. See also Carol C. Nadelson and Malkah T. Notman, "The Impact of the New Psychology of Men and Women on Psychotherapy," in *Review of Psychiatry*, ed. Allan Tasman and Stephen M. Goldfinger (Washington, D.C.: American Psychiatric Press, 1991), 608–26.

101. See Committee on Women to Robert Spitzer, July 12, 1979, *DSM* Files, Spitzer Papers, Melvin Sabshin Library and Archives, American Psychiatric Association, Washington, D.C.

102. See, for example, Walter R. Gove, "The Relationship between Sex Roles, Marital Status, and Mental Illness," *Social Forces* 51 (1972): 34–44; Lenore Radloff, "Sex Differences in Depression: The Effects of Occupation and Marital Status," *Sex Roles* 1 (1975): 249–65.

103. For a thoughtful, contemporary commentary on women's social roles and their interactions with psychiatry, see Virginia Abernethy, "Cultural Perspectives on the Impact of Women's Changing Roles on Psychiatry," *American Journal of Psychiatry* 133 (1976): 657–61.

104. Myrna M. Weissman and Gerald L. Klerman, "Sex Differences and the Epidemiology of Depression," *Archives of General Psychiatry* 34 (1977): 98–111.

105. George Winokur, Samuel B. Guze, and Eric Pfeiffer, "Developmental and Sexual Factors in Women: A Comparison between Control, Neurotic and Psychotic Groups," *American Journal of Psychiatry* 115 (1959): 1097–1100, quote from 1099–1100.

106. While some critical to psychoanalysis insisted that interpretations were somewhat rigid, feminist analyst Juliet Mitchell argued in the 1970s that psychoanalysis itself could actually be used for feminist purposes. Juliet Mitchell, *Psychoanalysis and Feminism* (New York: Pantheon Books, 1974).

107. Max Hamilton, "A Rating Scale for Depression," *Journal of Neurology, Neurosurgery and Psychiatry* 23 (1960): 56–62.

108. A. T. Beck et al., "An Inventory for Measuring Depression," *Archives of General Psychiatry* 4 (1961): 561–71. For Beck's description of Cognitive Behavioral Therapy (CBT), see Beck, *Cognitive Therapy and the Emotional Disorders*.

109. See, for example, William W. K. Zung, "A Cross-Cultural Survey of Symptoms in Depression," *American Journal of Psychiatry* 126 (1969): 116–21.

110. For the observation about the fit between the scales and the therapies they were designed to track, see Healy, *Antidepressant Era*, 98–99.

111. Max Hamilton, "Development of a Rating Scale for Primary Depressive Illness," *British Journal of Social and Clinical Psychology* 6 (1967): 278–96. Hamilton's scale is still used widely in depression research and has the benefit of being nonproprietary—it can be found easily (such as on the Internet) and can be used without need for permission or fees.

112. Beck and Beamesderfer, "Assessment of Depression." The BDI is still in clinical use, but it has been modified and trademarked, and now has to be purchased from the publisher in order to be used.

113. On constructions of masculinity over the twentieth century, see Michael S. Kimmel, *Manhood in America: A Cultural History* (New York: Free Press, 1996). A popular book on men's depression from the 1990s stresses that men's style is to not talk about their feelings. See Terrence Real, *I Don't Want to Talk About It: Overcoming the Secret Legacy of Male Depression* (New York: Fireside, 1997).

114. Feighner et al., "Hormonal Potentiation," 1231. The commentator's remarks were published at the end of the paper.
115. Feighner et al., "Hormonal Potentiation." For the diagnostic nomenclature officially recommended by the Washington University group, see Feighner et al., "Diagnostic Criteria for Use in Psychiatric Research," 57–63.
116. On Spitzer's emphasis on agreement—identified with the literature as reliability—see Kirk and Kutchins, *Selling of DSM*.
117. Spitzer, Endicott, and Robins, "Research Diagnostic Criteria."
118. American Psychiatric Association, *Diagnostic and Statistical Manual of Mental Disorders*, 3rd ed., 213–14.
119. Lee N. Robins and Darrel A. Regier, eds., *Psychiatric Disorders in America: The Epidemiologic Catchment Area Study* (New York: Free Press, 1991).
120. This assumption did not go entirely without comment, however. Jerome Myers and Myrna Weissman pointed out that people screened in population studies and patient studies might use self-rating scales differently. Jerome K. Myers and Myrna M. Weissman, "Use of a Self-Report Symptom Scale to Detect Depression in a Community Sample," *American Journal of Psychiatry* 137 (1980): 1081–84.
121. See Craig and Van Natta, "Presence and Persistence of Depressive Symptoms in Patient and Community Populations." One group of epidemiologists used the CES-D to survey married couples, but they had to do their analysis by disregarding the variables that were different between the men and the women. See Catherine E. Ross and John Mirowsky, "Components of Depressed Mood in Married Men and Women: The Center for Epidemiologic Studies' Depression Scale," *American Journal of Epidemiology* 119 (1984): 997–1004.
122. See, for example, Lino Covi, Ronald S. Lipman, Renato D. Alarcon, and Virginia K. Smith, "Drug and Psychotherapy Interactions in Depression," *American Journal of Psychiatry* 133 (1976): 502–8.
123. On the current significance of irritability for men's depression, see the epilogue.
124. See, for example, Candice J. Ranelli and Robert E. Miller, "Behavioral Predictors of Amitriptyline Response in Depression," *American Journal of Psychiatry* 138 (1981): 30–34.
125. Karen Beckman, Anthony J. Marsella, and Ruth Finney, "Depression in the Wives of Nuclear Submarine Personnel," *American Journal of Psychiatry* 136 (1979): 524–26.
126. Laura D. Hirshbein, "History of Women in Psychiatry," *Academic Psychiatry* 28 (2004): 337–43.
127. See, for example, Gabrielle A. Carlson and Diana C. Miller, "Suicide, Affective Disorder, and Women Physicians," *American Journal of Psychiatry* 138 (1981): 1330–35.
128. See, for example, Ellen Leibenluft, ed., *Gender Differences in Mood and Anxiety Disorders: From Bench to Bedside* (Washington, D.C.: American Psychiatric Press, 1999).
129. Kimmel, *Manhood in America*, 223–90. There has been increasing recognition of the fact that men in post—World War II America did not necessarily talk about their emotional experiences. Men who experienced traumatic wartime events, for example, did not discuss them at all (or not until many years later). See Robert Drury and Tom Clavin, *Halsey's Typhoon: The True Story of a Fighting Admiral, an Epic Storm, and an Untold Rescue* (New York: Grove Press, 2007).
130. On the controversy within the American psychiatric definition of homosexuality as

a mental illness, see Bayer, *Homosexuality and American Psychiatry*. Researchers who looked at men did not necessarily look for mental illness. Harvard psychiatrist George Valliant, for example, spent many years of his career assessing normal development in a group of college graduates—he tended to stress their adjustment rather than their pathologies. George E. Vaillant, "Why Men Seek Psychotherapy: I. Results of a Survey of College Graduates," *American Journal of Psychiatry* 129 (1972): 645–51; George E. Vaillant, "Natural History of Male Psychological Health: VI. Correlates of Successful Marriage and Fatherhood," *American Journal of Psychiatry* 135 (1978): 653–59; George E. Vaillant, "Natural History of Male Psychological Health: VIII. Antecedents of Alcoholism and 'Orality,'" *American Journal of Psychiatry* 137 (1980): 181–86; George E. Vaillant and Eva Milofsky, "Natural History of Male Psychological Health: IX. Empirical Evidence for Erikson's Model of the Life Cycle," *American Journal of Psychiatry* 137 (1980): 1348–59.

131. The few studies on depression in men generally included some attention to the issue of substance abuse. See, for example, John E. Hamm, Leslie F. Major, and Gerald L. Brown, "The Quantitative Measurement of Depression and Anxiety in Male Alcoholics," *American Journal of Psychiatry* 136 (1979): 580–82; Myrna M. Weissman and Jerome K. Myers, "Clinical Depression in Alcoholism," *American Journal of Psychiatry* 137 (1980): 372–73; Marc A. Schuckit, "Prevalence of Affective Disorder in a Sample of Young Men," *American Journal of Psychiatry* 139 (1982): 1431–36.

132. The MMPI was (and is) a psychologist-developed comprehensive assessment tool. On the history of the MMPI, see Roderick D. Buchanan, "The Development of the Minnesota Multiphasic Personality Inventory," *Journal of the History of the Behavioral Sciences* 30 (1994): 148–61.

133. Martin H. Keeler, C. Inga Taylor, and William C. Miller, "Are All Recently Detoxified Alcoholics Depressed?" *American Journal of Psychiatry* 136 (1979): 586–88.

134. William H. Hague, Lawrence G. Wilson, Donald L. Dudley, and Dale S. Cannon, "Post-Detoxification Drug Treatment of Anxiety and Depression in Alcohol Addicts," *Journal of Nervous and Mental Disease* 162 (1976): 354–59.

135. A few researchers in the 1980s raised questions about the extent to which changing social roles might affect psychiatric disease prevalence. See, for example, Ronnie S. Stangler and Adolph M. Printz, "*DSM-III*: Psychiatric Diagnosis in a University Population," *American Journal of Psychiatry* 137 (1980): 937–40; Ellen Frank, Linda L. Carpenter, and David J. Kupfer, "Sex Differences in Recurrent Depression: Are There Any That Are Significant?" *American Journal of Psychiatry* 145 (1988): 41–45.

136. Race is likely an important factor in the American construction of illness, though there is little primary or secondary literature on this topic. While researchers were eager to list the sex breakdown in their clinical trials, they almost never included race. Epidemiologists in the last several decades have explored how race might affect disease diagnosis distribution. James S. Jackson et al., "The National Survey of American Life: A Study of Racial, Ethnic and Cultural Influences on Mental Disorders and Mental Health," *International Journal of Methods in Psychiatric Research* 13 (2004): 196–207.

137. For a description of the emergence of another disease category that validates distress—post-traumatic distress disorder—see Young, *Harmony of Illusions*.

138. Janet B. W. Williams and Robert L. Spitzer, "The Issue of Sex Bias in *DSM-III*. A Critique of 'A Woman's View of *DSM-III*' by Marcie Kaplan," *American Psychologist*

38 (1983): 793–98; Robert L. Spitzer and Janet B. W. Williams, "Hysteroid Dysphoria: An Unsuccessful Attempt to Demonstrate Its Syndromal Validity," *American Journal of Psychiatry* 139 (1982): 1286–91.

139. *DSM-IV* was published in 1994. American Psychiatric Association, *Diagnostic and Statistical Manual of Mental Disorders*, 4th ed. (Washington, D.C.: American Psychiatric Association, 1994), 655–58.

140. Pamela Reed Gibson, "Histrionic Personality," in Caplan and Cosgrove, *Bias in Psychiatric Diagnosis*, 201–6, quote from 202.

141. Caplan, *They Say You're Crazy*, 122.

142. Laura Davidow Hirshbein, "Biology and Mental Illness: A Historical Perspective," *Journal of the American Medical Women's Association* 58 (2003): 89–94.

143. Not all feminists are critics of PMDD and personality disorders. On the complicated set of alliances and antagonisms around PMDD (formerly known as Late Luteul Phase Dysphoric Disorder [LLPDD]), see Anne E. Figert, "The Three Faces of PMS: The Professional, Gendered, and Scientific Structuring of a Psychiatric Disorder," *Social Problems* 42 (1995): 56–73.

144. Robins and Regier, *Psychiatric Disorders in America*. For current issues around gender in the treatment of depression from psychiatrists' point of view, see, for example, Kimberly A. Yonkers and Olga Brawman-Mintzer, "The Pharmacologic Treatment of Depression: Is Gender a Critical Factor?" *Journal of Clinical Psychiatry* 63 (2002): 610–15, Edyta J. Frackiewicz, John J. Sramek, and Neal R. Cutler, "Gender Differences in Depression and Antidepressant Pharmacokinetics and Adverse Events," *Annals of Pharmacotherapy* 34 (2000): 80–88.

145. One author argued that the *DSM* criteria might be biased *away* from women because they do not take into account women's social and cultural contexts that might encourage depression. Sarah McSweeney, "Depression in Women," in Caplan and Cosgrove, *Bias in Psychiatric Diagnosis*, 183–88.

146. See, for example, Carol S. Aneshensel, Ralph R. Frerichs, and Virginia A. Clark, "Family Roles and Sex Differences in Depression," *Journal of Health and Social Behavior* 22 (1981): 379–93.

147. See, for example, Joanne Steuer, Lew Bank, Edwin J. Olsen, and Lissy F. Jarvik, "Depression, Physical Health and Somatic Complaints in the Elderly: A Study of the Zung Self-Rating Depression Scale," *Journal of Gerontology* 35 (1980): 683–88.

148. A 1984 study from the University of California Irvine suggested that hospitalized depressed men and women had significantly different symptoms profiles. See Mark Zetin, Gloria Joy Sklansky, and Michelle Cramer, "Sex Differences in Inpatients with Major Depression," *Journal of Clinical Psychiatry* 45 (1984): 257–59. See also Melvin L. Selzer, Maria Paluszny, and Robert Carroll, "A Comparison of Depression and Physical Illness in Men and Women," *American Journal of Psychiatry* 135 (1978): 1368–70.

149. Issues of race in psychiatry have not been explored with nearly the rigor with they deserve. For an important account of how race affected psychiatric treatment primarily in the nineteenth-century South, see McCandless, *Moonlight, Magnolias, and Madness*. For a discussion of race and treatment during World War II, see Ellen Dwyer, "Psychiatry and Race during World War II," *Journal of the History of Medicine and Allied Sciences* 61 (2006): 117–43.

150. Monica D. Blumenthal, "Sex as a Source of Heterogeneity in a Mental Health Survey," *Journal of Psychiatric Research* 5 (1967): 75–87.

151. Ronald C. Kessler, Roger L. Brown, and Clifford Broman, "Sex Differences in

Psychiatric Help-Seeking: Evidence from Four Large-Scale Surveys," *Journal of Health and Social Behavior* 22 (1981): 49–64. A group in Switzerland also found that men may be more likely to forget times of depression, leading to bias using recalled symptoms in community studies. J. Angst and A. Dobler-Mikola, "Do the Diagnostic Criteria Determine the Sex Ratio in Depression?" *Journal of Affective Disorders* 7 (1984): 189–98.

152. See, for example, Andreasen and Winokur, "Newer Experimental Methods."

153. This is a sticky and confusing issue in the psychiatric literature. See, for example, Weissman and Myers, "Clinical Depression in Alcoholism"; Schuckit, "Prevalence of Affective Disorder."

154. On this point, see especially Horwitz, *Creating Mental Illness*; Horwitz and Wakefield, *Loss of Sadness*.

Chapter 5 — Feelings and Relationships

1. Senator Eagleton had been chosen by McGovern on July 13, 1972. The *New York Times* account of Eagleton, prior to the disclosure about his "nervous troubles," indicated that he was well respected and considered a good asset to the Democratic ticket. "McGovern Begins," *New York Times*, July 14, 1972.

2. James M. Naughton, "Eagleton Illness Known to Associates," *New York Times*, July 26, 1972.

3. Steven V. Roberts, "Messages of Support Sent to Eagleton," *New York Times*, August 1, 1972.

4. The public was not only concerned about Eagleton's history of depression but also his history of having received electroconvulsive therapy (ECT). See, for example, "Depression and Electroshock," *Newsweek*, August 7, 1972, 20; "The Most Common Mental Disorder," *Time*, August 7, 1972, 16; "Evaluating Eagleton," *Time*, August 14, 1972, 41. A sociological analysis completed a few years later pointed out that the media, not public opinion, were the decisive factor in Eagleton's forced resignation. Further, the media accounts were influenced by the fact that the period in which this happened was a slow news time and that the media did not know how to handle news reports about mental illness. David L. Altheide, "Mental Illness and the News: The Eagleton Story," *Sociology and Social Research* 61 (1977): 138–55. For an analysis of the rhetoric surrounding the media coverage of Eagleton, see Ernest G. Bormann, "The Eagleton Affair: A Fantasy Theme Analysis," *Quarterly Journal of Speech* 59 (1973): 143–59.

5. "McGovern Calls Eagleton Affair 'Saddest Part,'" *New York Times*, December 13, 1972. A psychoanalyst familiar only with the media reports of the case weighed in with his professional opinion shortly before Eagleton withdrew his candidacy. Mortimer Ostow, letter to the editor, *New York Times*, July 28, 1972. For a response to the psychoanalyst, see Murray Berman, letter to the editor, *New York Times*, August 4, 1972. For a psychiatric perspective a year later, see Willard Gaylin, "What's Normal?" *New York Times*, April 1, 1973.

6. The concept of anxiety was also an important one in the 1950s and 1960s. See Tone, *Age of Anxiety*.

7. For more on the magazine coverage of Eagleton's ECT treatment, see Hirshbein and Sarvananda, "History, Power, and Electricity."

8. For the growth and prevalence of consumer culture in the United States in the twentieth century, see Cohen, *Consumers' Republic*. See also Susan Strasser, ed.,

Commodifying Everything: Relationships of the Market (New York: Routledge, 2003).

9. There is an abundant literature on the psychology of stigma, but there is not much on the role of gender and stigma in mental illness. Todd F. Heatherton, Robert E. Kleck, Michelle R. Hebl, and Jay G. Hull, eds., *The Social Psychology of Stigma* (New York: Guilford Press, 2000).

10. Samuel McComb, "Nervousness in Women: Its Cause and Cure," *Harper's Bazar*, October 1907, 962–64, quote from 962. See also Samuel McComb, "Nervous Miseries and How to Fight Them," *Harper's Bazar*, August 1908, 719–21.

11. Maud Howe, "Nerves," *Harper's Bazar*, November 1908, 1136–38; George Lincoln Walton, "Those Nerves: Character-Leakage," *Lippincott's Magazine*, September 1909, 363–65; George Lincoln Walton, "Those Nerves: Sidetractibility," *Lippincott's Magazine*, August 1909, 202–4; John B. Huber, "A Shoddy Nervous System," *Collier's*, November 13, 1915, 32; Samuel McComb, "Work and Its Healing Power," *Harper's Bazar*, February 1909, 122–24.

12. John K. Mitchell, "Self Help for Nervous Women," *Harper's Bazar*, September 1901, 409–11, quote from 411.

13. Charles Phelps Cushing, "The Business Man with 'Nerves,'" *World's Work*, September 1916, 569–74, quote from 572. Cushing's article was advertised as being sanctioned by the Life Extension Institute, a private agency devoted to trying to improve the health and efficiency of businessmen. See Laura Davidow Hirshbein, "Masculinity, Work, and the Fountain of Youth: Irving Fisher and the Life Extension Institute: 1914–31," *Canadian Bulletin of Medical History* 16 (1999): 89–124.

14. Emotion in this case included violent anger. See Stanley M. Rinehart, "Your Nerves and Your Job," *Saturday Evening Post*, February 19, 1921, 14–15, 68–70.

15. On the growing prevalence of psychological language in the United States in the years after World War II, see Herman, *Romance of American Psychology*.

16. Mary Ellen Zuckerman, *A History of Popular Women's Magazines in the United States, 1792–1995* (Westport, Conn.: Greenwood Press, 1998).

17. See Frank J. McGowan, "The Doctor Talks About Postnatal Blues," *McCall's*, June 1957, 4, 143; Frank J. McGowan, "The Doctor Talks About Depression," *McCall's*, May 1958, 4, 151–53; "Those Mysterious Childbirth Blues," *Good Housekeeping*, May 1960, 165–66.

18. Sprague H. Gardiner, "The Expectant Mother," *Redbook*, October 1967, 31–32, quote from 31. See also Yanna Kroyt Brandt, "What Doctors Now Know About Depressed Young Mothers," *Redbook*, March 1968, 68–69, 162–65; Shirley G. Streshinsky, "The Truth About Those New Mother Blues," *Parents Magazine*, April 1969, 56–57, 64–66.

19. See, for example, Hollan, "Depression Is the Pits"; L.H., "How to Tell if You're Depressed," *Good Housekeeping*, March 1989, 209.

20. Kelley Massoni, "'Teena Goes to Market': *Seventeen* Magazine and the Early Construction of the Teen Girl as Consumer," *Journal of American Culture* 29 (2006): 31–42.

21. There was little attention in this period to depressed adolescent boys, and boys did not have the same publishing machine directed toward marketing reading material for them. For one account of a boy's depression and suicide attempt (from his mother's point of view), see "My Son Tried to Kill Himself," *Good Housekeeping*, May 1987, 30–34.

22. "10 Ways to Beat the Blues." See also "Teenage Depression"; "Dealing with Depression." One 1986 article used celebrities to provide suggestions for teenagers on how they could help themselves feel better. "What Stars Do to Shine."

23. De Rosis and Pellegrino, "Depression on the Job," 129. See also "Jog Away Depression," *Harper's Bazaar*, January 1979, 113.

24. Banashek, "Depression." Teenagers were also encouraged not to wallow in their depression, but rather to fight it. See, for example, Kathy McCoy, "Getting Over the Breakup Blues," *Seventeen*, March 1987, 34, 38; "In the Dumps? 10 Easy Picker Uppers," *Teen*, November 1989, 52, 100.

25. David Smith, "How to Exercise Your Way Out of a Depression," *Mademoiselle*, April 1979, 194, 234–36; "Exercise Plus"; Numata, "Lifting Weights and Spirits"; Stark, "Exercising Away Depression," 68; Spilner, "Taking the High Road"; "Don't Just Sit There."

26. See, for example, Klein, "Running Away from Depression," 85. A 1985 article in *Prevention* (by a male psychiatrist) advocated running for women to help them achieve a sense of mastery. William Gottlieb, "Headstrong: Exercise as Therapy," *Prevention*, July 1985, 61–63.

27. Ellen Frank and David J. Kupfer, "The Battle against the Blues," *Ladies' Home Journal*, March 1985, 147–54.

28. For an analysis of women's views of body sizes in the twentieth century, see Joan Jacobs Brumberg, *The Body Project: An Intimate History of American Girls* (New York: Random House, 1997); Peter N. Stearns, *Fat History: Bodies and Beauty in the Modern West* (New York: New York University Press, 1997).

29. "Smile! The Mood Makeover," *Mademoiselle*, December 1990, 172–75, quote from 173, ellipses in the original.

30. Wayne's assertion was listed among a group of celebrities in their reports of what they do when they are feeling blue. "How I Beat the Blues," 90–91. For an analysis of twentieth-century masculinity, especially the way in which figures such as John Wayne fit in, see Kimmel, *Manhood in America*. For the stresses within Cold War masculinity in particular, see Cuordileone, *Manhood and American Political Culture in the Cold War*.

31. Storr, "Winston Churchill's Black Dog."

32. Knauth, "Season in Hell." See also Stoler, "Season in Hell."

33. "William Styron," *People*, December 31, 1990, 86; William Styron, *Darkness Visible: A Memoir of Madness* (New York: Random House, 1990).

34. Hutschnecker, "If You're Depressed."

35. Competition with women could also lead to depression, as evidenced by an account of Prince Claus of Denmark, who became depressed in part because he had difficulty with the fact that his wife, the queen, enjoyed the spotlight. Wibo van de Linde, "His Strength Exhausted, Holland's Prince Claus Is Hospitalized for Severe Depression," *People*, November 1, 1982, 107.

36. Ellen Goodman, "Why Men Feel Like Failures and Women Don't," *McCall's*, November 1979, 236.

37. Sandy Keenan, "'I Wasn't a Normal Person': Severe Depression Nearly Destroyed Brad Cochran of Michigan," *Sports Illustrated*, October 14, 1985, 83–84; "Depression Almost Killed Ex-Manager Maury Wills."

38. Tevis, "Depression"; "Personal Management," *Successful Farming*, March 1984, 22AO.

39. Maynard, "Even Winners Battle the Blues."

40. Stein, "Rising Above Malaise."

41. For historical perspective on the problems with men and feelings, see Mary Chapman and Glenn Hendler, eds., *Sentimental Men: Masculinity and the Politics of Affect in American Culture* (Berkeley: University of California Press, 1999).

42. On changes in women's roles over time, see Sheila M. Rothman, *Woman's Proper Place: A History of Changing Ideals and Practices, 1870 to the Present* (New York: Basic Books, 1978).

43. Abraham Myerson, "The Nervous Housewife," *Ladies' Home Journal*, November 1920, 26–27, 132–38, quote from 27.

44. "Our Perilous Waste of Vitality," *Literary Digest*, April 27, 1912, 878–79, quote from 878. See also Max G. Schlapp, "The Enemy at the Gate," *Outlook*, April 6, 1912, 782–88.

45. See, for example, "Increasing Insanity," *Current Literature*, May 1904, 547–48.

46. "The Need of Rational Thinking," *Independent*, May 26, 1923, 330.

47. Edward H. Smith, "The Reds and the Glands," *Saturday Evening Post*, August 21, 1920, 6–7, 162–70. In 1932, the *New Republic* reported that a former student of the University of Wisconsin was committed to an asylum because of his political beliefs. Fortunately, according to the article, the asylum staff found nothing wrong with him and released him after six days. "Political Insanity," *New Republic*, August 17, 1932, 7.

48. See especially May, *Homeward Bound*. See also Jane F. Levey, "Imagining the Family in Postwar Popular Culture: The Case of *The Egg and I* and *Cheaper By the Dozen*," *Journal of Women's History* 13 (2001): 125–50. For the long view on changes in marital structures, including the more recent emphasis on intimacy within marriage, see Stephanie Coontz, *Marriage, a History: From Obedience to Intimacy or How Love Conquered Marriage* (New York: Viking, 2005).

49. See, for example, "The New Depression Treatments," *Harper's Bazaar*, September 1973, 159, 168; R. W. Shepherd, "Is Your Depression a Real Tiger?" *Vogue*, June 1978, 111–13.

50. For example, Myrna Weissman pointed out in 1972 that women experienced conflicts because, even though they were working in greater numbers, they were still vulnerable to being moved around because of their husband's job. Myrna M. Weissman and Eugene S. Paykel, "Moving and Depression in Women," *Society*, July–August 1972, 24–28.

51. Kathleen Brady, "Does Liberation Cause Depression?" *Harper's Bazaar*, February 1976, 118–19; Elizabeth Howard, "Even Superwomen Get the Blues," *Working Woman*, January 1980, 51–52; Maureen Smith Williams, "Monday: The Worst Morning of All," *McCall's*, August 1982, 45.

52. De Rosis and Pellegrino, "Depression on the Job"; Helen A. DeRosis and Victoria Y. Pellegrino, *The Book of Hope: How Women Can Overcome Depression* (New York: Bantam, 1977).

53. Marie Saunders, "Depression: The Blues Within," *Essence*, April 1980, 91, 134–39.

54. Hamilton, "Are You Blue?" See also Nevada Harris Mitchell, "Hope for Depression," *Essence*, June 1988, 16, 132.

55. Maggie Scarf, *Unfinished Business: Pressure Points in the Lives of Women* (New York: Doubleday, 1980). Scarf continued to be an authority on depression in popular magazines in the years after her book no longer gathered headlines. See, for example, Maggie Scarf and Myrna M. Weissman, "Shades of Blue . . ." *McCall's*, July 1984, 66.

56. For popular articles based on her book, see Maggie Scarf, "Women and Depression," *New Republic*, July 5, 1980, 25–29; Maggie Scarf, "Women Depressed—Why?" *Vogue*, August 1980, 255, 283–84; Patricia Bosworth, "Emotional Passages of Women," *Working Woman*, February 1981, 84–90.

57. For commentary about feminist responses to Scarf's book, see Cynthia H. Wilson and Eric Gruman, "Why Women Are Depressed," *Newsweek*, September 8, 1980, 81–82.

58. Scarf's views made so much sense at the time that they were used to explain the unthinkable—a woman who became depressed and killed herself and her small children. Scarf explained that this was due to the woman's sense of connection to her children, that she was suffering so much that she believed that they were suffering, too. Linda Wolfe, "A Tragedy on 89th Street," *New York*, October 20, 1980, 41–47.

59. For historians' descriptions of women's social networks and culture in the past, see, for example, Carroll Smith-Rosenberg, *Disorderly Conduct: Visions of Gender in Victorian America* (New York: Alfred A. Knopf, 1985); Estelle Freedman, "Separatism as Strategy: Female Institution Building and American Feminism, 1870–1930," *Feminist Studies* 5 (1979): 512–29; Mary Ryan, *Womanhood in America from Colonial Times to the Present*, 2nd ed. (New York: Viewpoints, 1983); Morantz-Sanchez, *Sympathy and Science*.

60. See, for example, Karen Lindsey, "Rx for Depression: One Friend Every 4 Hours," *Ms.*, June 1979, 57–59.

61. Harriet B. Braiker, "Why Depression Is Different for High-Achieving Women," *Working Woman*, December 1987, 79–83.

62. Psychologist Phyllis Chesler argued in 1972 that physicians over the centuries had labeled women as mentally ill in order to gain control over them. Chesler, *Women and Madness*. Maggie Scarf explicitly refuted Chesler, though, saying that depression was part of women's biological heritage, not the result of labeling. Judy Gould, "Expert Maggie Scarf Finds That Depression Afflicts Up to Six Times More U.S. Women Than Men," *People*, September 15, 1980, 107–10. For more on the relationship between popular culture and the feminist movement in this time period, see Sherrie A. Inness, ed., *Disco Divas: Women and Popular Culture in the 1970s* (Philadelphia: University of Pennsylvania Press, 2003).

63. Ann Thacher-Renshaw and Carol Goldberg Kirsch, "When the New Mother Blues Go On . . . and On . . . and On," *Parents Magazine*, February 1978, 16–17, 34. See also "Support Groups for New Moms," *Changing Times*, November 1981, 52.

64. "Postbirth Blues," *Time*, March 10, 1980, 58.

65. Lake, "How to Cope"; M.L.S., "New Ways to Spot and Treat Depression," 205; Norwood, "Great Depression."

66. See Robert L. Griswold, *Fatherhood in America: A History* (New York: Basic Books, 1993).

67. Ann Slegman, "Color Father Blue," *McCall's*, June 1982, 52; Ross Wetzsteon, "Why Fathers Get the New-Baby Blues," *Redbook*, July 1983, 19, 24.

68. Myrna M. Weissman, "Men and Depression," *Glamour*, May 1980, 142–45.

69. Sonya Friedman, "Why Husbands—and All of Us—Get the Holiday Blues, and How to Cope," *Ladies' Home Journal*, December 1984, 72.

70. Moskowitz, "How to Live with His Worst Moods."

71. Dianne Hales, "When Your Husband Is Depressed," *McCall's*, May 1986, 38–40.

72. Knox, "Blues Really Get You Down."

73. Friedan, *Feminine Mystique*. For the movement's exhortations for collective action, see Sara M. Evans, *Personal Politics: The Roots of Women's Liberation in the Civil Rights Movement and the New Left* (New York: Knopf, 1979).

74. Lears, "From Salvation to Self-Realization."

75. Anna Sturges Duryea, "Making Friends of One's Nerves," *Delineator*, June 1909, 774, 820–21, quote from 774.

76. Agnes Repplier, "The Nervous Strain," *Atlantic Monthly*, August 1910, 198–201. For an analysis of early-twentieth-century nostalgia, see Lears, *No Place of Grace*.

77. For a critique of the ways in which the mythical savage environment shaped sociologists' and biologists' assumptions about sex and gender, see Ruth Bleier, *Science and Gender: A Critique of Biology and Its Theories on Women* (New York: Pergamon Press, 1984).

78. "Nerve Diseases Caused by Success in Life," *Current Opinion*, December 1918, 380.

79. Samuel McComb, "Nerves in the Home," *Harper's Bazar*, July 1910, 468.

80. "Nervous and Emotional States Not Inherited," *Current Opinion*, November 1918, 309–10.

81. Annie Payson Call, "Why Does Mrs. Smith Get on My Nerves?" *Ladies' Home Journal*, September 1908, 22.

82. Harvey W. Wiley, "The Best Cure for Nervousness," *Good Housekeeping*, October 1925, 86–92, 318–23, quote from 318. On Harvey Wiley's career with the Food and Drug Administration, see Jack C. High and Clayton Anderson Copping, *The Politics of Purity: Harvey Washington Wiley and the Origins of Federal Food Policy* (Ann Arbor: University of Michigan Press, 1999).

83. See Call, *Power through Repose*.

84. McCall, "Girl Who Is Nervous."

85. Narratives of nervousness reinforced concurrent popular exhortations for women to improve their health through proper clothing and exercise. See Martha H. Verbrugge, "Recreating the Body: Women's Physical Education and the Science of Sex Differences in America, 1900–1940," *Bulletin of the History of Medicine* 71 (1997): 273–304. On beauty standards of the time, see Lois W. Banner, *American Beauty* (Chicago: University of Chicago Press, 1983).

86. Anonymous, "The Autobiography of a Neurasthenic," *American Magazine*, December 1910, 223–31, quote from 231. It is probably not a coincidence that this man, who criticized the American drive in men, refused to attach his own name to the article.

87. Graham, "To Beat the Blues." Graham's article was condensed from *Redbook*.

88. Richard Camer, "Dressed for Depression," *Psychology Today*, January 1985, 70.

89. "79 Surefire Ways to Pick Yourself Up When You're Down and Out," *Mademoiselle*, April 1974, 172–75; Viorst, "How to Feel Better When You're Feeling Rotten."

90. Catherine Findlay, "15 Ways to Weather the Winter Blues," *Mademoiselle*, February 1983, 30–32; "20 Things Not to Do When You're Feeling Blue," *Glamour*, September 1985, 45; Kessler, "What to Do When You're Melancholy," 48.

91. "New Ways to Treat Depression." This article featured the opinions of Gerald Klerman. Critics of medication understood that physician advocates for drug treatments were attempting to sell them to the public as the only treatments for depression (as opposed to psychoanalysis). See Steck, "Drugs for Depression's

Sadness." For an enthusiastic pitch for structured therapy, see Beck and Kovacs, "New, Fast Therapy for Depression." For physician accounts of the range of options for women, see Hirschfeld, "Clinical Depression."

92. "Depression!"; Jabs, "Depressed?" In addition to medications, women also discussed the consumption of self-help books. See Marks, "What's Normal, What's Not?"

93. Goldman, "How to Cope."

94. Rodgers, "Christmas Depression Syndrome"; Lasswell and Lobsenz, "Living Happily through the Holidays." The enthusiasm for continued purchase was particularly striking during the late 1970s during a time of significant economic recession.

95. Etzioni, "Christmas Blues."

96. See, for example, Diane de Dubovay, "Coping with Christmas Blues," *Harper's Bazaar*, December 1978, 162, 196.

97. See, for example, Frank Trippett, "Get This Season Off the Couch!" *Time*, December 11, 1978, 130; "Good Listening," 40.

98. See, for example, Roth, "Anti-Depression Diet"; Jacoby, "When 'Joyful' Occasions Get You Down"; Bruns, "Sunday Blues"; Moramarco, "Food Blues?" Even *Ms.* magazine was not above offering advice to help with moods. Klein, "Running Away from Depression."

99. See, for example, Elizabeth Wurtzel, *Prozac Nation* (New York: Riverhead Books, 1994).

100. Jonathan V. Wright, "A Case of Apathy and Depression," *Prevention*, June 1984, 113–18.

101. Leonore Fleischer, "A Twist of Fate," *Publishers Weekly*, August 10, 1984, 79.

102. Linda Marx, "I Was Full of Terror and Fright," *People*, January 12, 1987, 35–36.

103. Kim Hubbard, "William Styron," *People*, August 27, 1990, 62–65.

104. Occasionally, men were offered advice about consumption in order to prevent emotional distress. One *Business Week* article commented that executives were always upset during the holiday season, partly because they had postponed their gift purchasing until very late. They were advised to plan ahead (although it was not clear that they were actually going to be the ones doing the early purchasing). See Hitchings, "How to Shake Those Holiday Blues."

105. Slovinsky, "Out of Depression," 36.

106. Andrew Solomon's more recent depression account echoes some of Slovinsky's themes. Solomon, *Noonday Demon.*

107. Stein, "Rising Above Malaise," 36. See also Harry Stein, *Ethics and Other Liabilities: Trying to Live Right in an Amoral World* (New York: St. Martin's Griffin, 1983).

108. For the specific cultural effects of Prozac by the 1990s, see, for example, Kramer, *Listening to Prozac*; Elizabeth Wurtzel, "Tangled Up in Blues," *Mademoiselle*, April 1990, 228–29, 260–61; Wurtzel, *Prozac Nation.*

109. Buckley, "You Can Beat Depression," 173.

Epilogue

1. NIMH, "Real Men. Real Depression." (2003), http://menanddepression.nimh.nih. gov, accessed April 28, 2007.

2. NIMH, "Real Men. Real Depression." brochure, 27–28, http://menanddepression. nimh.nih.gov, accessed April 28, 2007.

3. Some books intended for popular audiences have also pointed out the extent to which men have been left out of a consideration of depression. See, for example, Real, *I Don't Want to Talk About It*; Sam V. Cochran and Fredric E. Rabinowitz, *Men*

and Depression: Clinical and Empirical Perspectives (San Diego, Calif.: Academic Press, 2000).

4. "Real Men. Real Depression." brochure, 3.

5. Julie Scelfo, Karen Springen, and Mary Carmichael, "Men & Depression: Facing Darkness," *Newsweek*, February 26, 2007, 42–49.

6. Of course, the fact that cancer is held up as the prototypical disease to fight reflects a different, historically contingent process. See James T. Patterson, *The Dread Disease: Cancer and Modern American Culture* (Cambridge, Mass.: Harvard University Press, 1987).

7. The *Newsweek* article also included symptoms of alcohol abuse and acting out violently. Scelfo, Springen, and Carmichael, "Men & Depression."

8. Researchers who are currently exploring depression in older African Americans have noted that men are significantly less interested in the label of depression, even to describe the same symptoms. Helen Kales, "The Impact of Race on the Diagnosis and Treatment of Depression," University of Michigan Department of Psychiatry, January 23, 2008. Note also that physical symptoms were much more prominent in the Hamilton depression scale—the one that was developed in an all-male patient population. Hamilton, "Rating Scale for Depression."

9. Constance Burr, "NIMH Launches 'Real Men. Real Depression.' Campaign," May 27, 2003, http://www.nih.gov/news/NIH-Record/05_27_2003/story03.htm, accessed April 28, 2007.

10. Jeffrey Kluger, "Real Men Get the Blues," *Time*, September 22, 2003, 48–49.

11. Scelfo, Springen, and Carmichael, "Men & Depression," 45.

12. In 2001, psychologist Gary Brooks explored some of the implications of definitions of mental health and illness and the changing nature of masculinity. He pointed out that many features of traditional ideas about masculinity—particularly violence, sexual misconduct, and substance abuse—worsen men's mental health overall and lead to increased likelihood of mental illness. Brooks argues that men need to be helped not just by understanding the ways in which masculine ideas and culture affect men in their mental health and illness, but also that cultural norms need to change to improve mental health. Gary R. Brooks, "Masculinity and Men's Mental Health," *Journal of American College Health* 49 (2001): 285–97.

13. Recent popular magazines have occasionally noted this problem of failure to accept unhappiness as part of our general human range of emotions. This has not been enough to slow pharmaceutical sales, however. See, for example, Sharon Begley, "Happiness: Enough Already," *Newsweek*, February 11, 2008, 50–52.

14. Jonathan Metzl has reflected on the dilemma of facing a patient who has come in with a specific medication request based on a direct-to-consumer advertisement. Jonathan M. Metzl, "Angela," *American Journal of Psychiatry* 159 (2002): 1665–66.

15. Kramer, *Listening to Prozac.*

16. See Carl Elliott, *Better Than Well: American Medicine Meets the American Dream* (New York: W. W. Norton, 2003); Carl Elliott and Tod Chambers, eds., *Prozac as a Way of Life* (Chapel Hill: University of North Carolina Press, 2004).

17. See, for example, Ronald Pies, "Redefining Depression as Mere Sadness," *New York Times*, September 16, 2008.

18. See A. John Rush et al., "Acute and Longer-Term Outcomes in Depressed Outpatients Requiring One or Several Treatment Steps: A STAR*D Report," *American Journal of Psychiatry* 163 (2006): 1905–17; Madhukar H. Trivedi et al., "Evaluation

of Outcomes with Citalopram for Depression Using Measurement-Based Care in STAR*D: Implications for Clinical Practice," *American Journal of Psychiatry* 163 (2006): 28–40.

19. Joan Jacobs Brumberg, *Fasting Girls: The Emergence of Anorexia Nervosa as a Modern Disease* (Cambridge, Mass.: Harvard University Press, 1988).

20. Robert A. Woodruff Jr., Paula Clayton, and Samuel B. Guze, "Is Everyone Depressed?" *American Journal of Psychiatry* 132 (1975): 627–28, quote from 628.

21. A recent explanation of global issues of depression authored by well-respected psychiatrists made many assertions, most of which were supported only by American data. The authors did not address the economics, treatment, and workforce issues for other countries. Philip S. Wang and Ronald C. Kessler, "Global Burden of Mood Disorders," in Stein, Kupfer, and Schatzberg, *American Psychiatric Publishing Textbook of Mood Disorders*, 55–67.

22. L. Staner and J. Mendlewicz, "Methodological Issues in Collaborative Multicenter Placebo-Controlled Studies in the Treatment of Depression," in *Critical Issues in the Treatment of Affective Disorders*, ed. S. Z. Langer et al. (Basel: Karger, 1994), 37–43.

23. Laurence J. Kirmayer and G. Eric Jarvis, "Depression Across Cultures," in Stein, Kupfer, and Schatzberg, *American Psychiatric Publishing Textbook of Mood Disorders*, 699–715.

24. Elizabeth Lunbeck has pointed out that psychiatry and psychoanalysis have contributed to the problem of American identity. Elizabeth Lunbeck, "Borderline Histories: Psychoanalysis Inside and Out," *Science in Context* 19 (2006): 151–73.

Index

5-HIAA, 47–48

adjustment, language of, 83
African American women, 115
Akiskal, Hagop, 47
alcoholism, 10, 40, 42, 48, 88–90, 92–93, 98, 101, 104
Aldrin, Edwin (Buzz), Jr., 123
allopathic treatment, 12
American Board of Psychiatry and Neurology, 14
Americanitis, 22–23, 119
American Neurological Association, 15
American Psychiatric Association, 15, 41, 44, 49, 102–103; Committee on Women, 95
American Psychological Association, 41–42
amphetamines, 46
Andreasen, Nancy, 43, 70
antipsychiatry, 132
anxiety, 16, 25, 44, 53–54, 57, 59, 107
Arieti, Silvano, 49
assessment tools, 31, 34–35, 38. *See also* rating scales

Babcock, Warren, 80
Ballentine, E. P., 82
Barker, Lewellys, 13
Barton, Walter, 33, 39
Beard, George M., 12
Beck, Aaron, 37, 66, 68, 97, 122
Beck Depression Inventory (BDI), 96–97
Beers, Clifford, 21
Bemporad, Jules, 49
bias, 7, 31, 95, 102–104
blues, 13, 64–65, 74, 110, 120–121
Blumenthal, Monica, 104
Bosselman, Beulah, 84
Braiker, Harriet, 116
Brothers, Joyce, 68
Brown, Bertram, 60–61, 72
Brumberg, Joan Jacobs, 130

Burns, David, 66
business issues, 5, 57

Call, Annie Payson, 120
Caplan, Paula, 103
Carroll, Bernard, 43, 48
case reports, 31–34
catecholamine hypothesis, 46–47
Center for Epidemiologic Studies Depression Scale (CES-D), 99
chemical imbalance, 62, 113
childbirth blues, 64, 110, 117
children, 69, 72–73
chlorpromazine (Thorazine), 29
Chodoff, Paul, 54
Churchill, Winston, 63, 70, 112, 123
classification. *See* nosology
Clayton, Paula, 131
Cognitive Behavioral Therapy (CBT), 37, 66, 97, 122
Cole, Jonathan, 27
Collaborative Depression Studies Program. *See under* National Institute of Mental Health
collective action, 116, 118, 122, 131
common cold of mental illness, 27, 68
Commonwealth Fund, 15
computer assessment, 39, 55
consent, 31
cortisol, 48

D'Agostino, Anthony, 47
de Kruif, Paul, 23
dementia praecox. *See* schizophrenia
depression, as economic condition, 1, 9, 58–60
depression, as mental condition: endogenous, 35–36, 43; exogenous (reactive), 35–36, 43; neurotic, 43; seasonal, 63, 67; symptoms, 3, 27–28, 32, 42, 44–45
Depression Awareness, Recognition, and Treatment campaign (NIMH), 52

Depression for Dummies (Smith and Elliott), 76
Dercum, Francis, 80
DeRosis, Helen, 111
dexamethasone suppression test (DST), 43, 48
diagnosis, valid, 38, 40, 55
Diagnostic and Statistical Manual (*DSM*); *DSM-I*, 38; *DSM-II*, 5, 39–40; *DSM-III*, 2, 40–46, 49–50, 54, 61, 95–99; *DSM-IIIR*, 45–46, 100; *DSM-IV*, 128; *DSM-IV-TR*, 3, 103; *DSM-V*, 55, 132
diethyl stilbestrol (DES), 85
direct-to-consumer (DTC) advertising, 58, 122
double depression, 51
dysthymia, 51, 73

Eagleton, Thomas, 60, 107–108, 123
eating disorders, 130–131
educational campaigns, 3–4, 51–52
efficiency, 80, 109
electroconvulsive therapy (ECT), 15, 22–23, 29–30, 87–89, 98, 108, 121
Ellison, Harlan, 122
Emerson, Haven, 15
Emmanuel Movement, 20–21, 109
Endicott, Jean, 34, 39
endogenous depression, 35–36, 43
Epidemiological Catchment Area (ECA) Study, 50, 99
epidemiology, 28, 49–51, 53, 55, 59, 99, 103
estrogen, 2, 92–93
eugenics, 22–23
exercise, 64, 67, 111
exogenous (reactive) depression, 35–36, 43

Farrar, Clarence, 13, 85
Faust, David, 55
Feighner, John, 40, 54, 98
Feighner criteria, 40–41, 55, 98
feminist movement, 94–95, 116–118, 122, 131
fluoxetine. *See* Prozac
Food and Drug Administration (FDA), 4
Franks, Ruth MacLachlan, 85
Freud, Sigmund, 14, 24
Freyhan, Fritz, 90
Friedan, Betty, 94–95, 118

Gardner, Sprague, 110
genetics, 36,48
Gibson, Pamela Reed, 102
Gittelman, Rachel, 42
Goode, Erica, 75–76
Goodman, Ellen, 112
Griesinger, Wilhelm, 11
Guze, Samuel, 40, 131
gynecology, 82

Hamilton, Max, 96–97
Hamilton Depression Scale (HDS), 96–97, 101
Hazleton, Lesley, 74–75
Healy, David, 27, 54
Hippocrates, 9
Hirschfeld, Robert, 74–75
histrionic personality disorder, 102
Hoch, August, 84
Hohman, Leslie, 15
homosexuality, 5, 40, 84, 100
Hopper, Edward, *Automat*, 3
hormones, 77, 82, 84–87, 93, 98
hospitals, psychiatric, 10–13, 23–24, 28–29, 31, 33, 89–92
Huston, Paul, 88
hysteria, 11, 40, 81–82

imipramine, 29–30, 32, 93, 98
immigrants, 22
insanity, 6, 12, 17–19, 21–25, 59, 77, 81, 113–114
insulin coma, 15, 23–24
Interpersonal Psychotherapy (IPT), 37, 66, 91
introjected aggression, 14
involutional melancholia, 2, 79, 81–87, 89
iproniazid (Marsalid), 29–31, 46
irritability, 45, 100, 128
isocarbazid, 32

Jackson, Stanley, 7–8
Jamison, Kay, 70
Jelliffe, Smith Ely, 11, 79
Jones, Ernest, 80

Katz, Martin, 36
Keller, Martin, 51
Kinsey, Alfred, 5

Klaiber, Edward, 92–93
Klein, Donald, 42, 47
Klerman, Gerald, 36, 43, 61, 68–69, 91
Kline, Nathan, 61, 65–66, 70, 73–74
Knauth, Percy, 61–62, 112, 117
Kraepelin, Emil, 11, 81
Kramer, Peter, 58, 130
Kupfer Detre Scale (KDS-3A), 34

Lincoln, Abraham, 63, 122
Linn, Erwin, 31
lithium, 34, 49
lobotomy, 15
Lochler, Lillian, 88

MacCoy, Cecil, 10–11
MacCurdy, John, 84
manic-depressive psychosis, 2, 11, 14–15,
    29, 38, 80–82, 84, 88–89
McComb, Samuel, 21, 109
McGovern, George, 60, 107
Menninger, Karl, 21
Menninger, Roy, 72
Menninger, William, 93–94
menopause, 63, 81, 84–87, 92
mental hospitals. *See* hospitals, psychiatric
mental hygiene, 17, 20–22, 79, 81
metrazol, 15, 23–24, 86
M.F. (masculinity/femininity) test, 84
MHPG, 47
Miles, Catherine, 84
Miltown, 54
Mind That Found Itself, A (Beers), 21
Miner, Richard, 55
Minnesota Multiphasic Personality
    Inventory (MMPI), 101
Mitchell, John, 109
Mitchell, S. Weir, 80
monoamine oxidase inhibitors (MAOIs), 32,
    46, 48, 62, 66–67, 92
Mourning and Melancholia (Freud), 14
Munoz, Rodrigo, 40
Myerson, Abraham, 114

narcosynthesis, 19
National Conference on Nomenclature of
    Disease, 15
National Institute of Mental Health
    (NIMH), 61, 63, 127, 132; Collaborative

Depression Studies Program, 36, 41, 51–
    52; "Real Men" campaign, 127–129
nervousness, 17–18, 20–25, 113–115
neurasthenia, 11–12, 17–18, 22, 79, 120
neurologists, 10–16, 24, 77–81, 100
neuroses, 3, 60, 109, 129
neurotic depression, 43
neurotransmitters, 46–48, 62–63, 92
New York Academy of Medicine, 15
New York State Psychiatric Institute, 36,
    40, 98
nialamide, 32
norepinephrine, 46–47
nosology, 15–16, 36, 54

older adults, 70
orphenadrine, 29

Papanicolaou, George, 87
Paton, Stewart, 114
Pellegrino, Victoria, 111
pep pill, 57
pharmaceutical companies, 4–5, 8, 28, 37,
    85
pharmaceutical industry, 6, 56, 58, 105, 132
phenelzine, 32
pheniprazine, 32
Pilgrim, Charles, 11
placebo-controlled trial, 31–32
Pollack, Benjamin, 30
Pollack, Horatio, 80–81
positron emission tomography (PET), 128
postpartum depression, 117. *See also*
    childbirth blues
Pratt, George, 21
Premenstrual Dysphoric Disorder (PMDD),
    102–103
primary care physicians, 50–51, 132
Prozac (fluoxetine), 4, 37, 51, 58, 67, 91,
    122–123, 130
psychiatric hospitals. *See* hospitals,
    psychiatric
psychiatrists: biologically oriented, 33–37;
    psychoanalytically oriented, 16, 24, 33–
    35, 42, 49, 54, 80–81, 83, 93; women, 100
psychoanalysis, 14, 24, 66, 79
psychology, 83–84; language of, 60, 94, 110
psychotherapy, 3, 12, 34, 37, 61, 66–67, 70,
    75–76, 111, 121–122

Raskin, Allen, 35
rating scales, 34–35, 38, 50, 101
reactive depression. *See* exogenous
    depression
Reagan, Ronald, 69
"Real Men. Real Depression." campaign.
    See under National Institute of Mental
    Health
reliability, 34, 38–40, 53, 55
Research Diagnostic Criteria (RDC), 40–42,
    44, 50, 55, 98
Rifkin, Arthur, 42
Ripley, Herbert, 87
Robie, Theodore (T.R.), 30, 46–47
Robins, Eli, 40

Sacher, Edward, 42
Sadler, William, 22–23
Saunders, Eleanora, 83
Saunders, Marie, 115
Scarf, Maggie, 116, 118
Schildkraut, Joseph, 46–47
schizophrenia, 15, 24–25, 29–30, 32, 37, 40,
    84, 89, 91
Schlapp, Max, 114
Schopbach, Robert, 31
Schuyler, Dean, 93
seasonal depression, 63, 67
Season in Hell, A (Knauth), 117
selective serotonin reuptake inhibitors
    (SSRIs), 4, 130
selective service screening, 19–20
self-help, 63–64, 67, 69, 76, 121, 123
Seligman, Martin, 74–75
serotonin, 46–47
Sheehy, Michael, 42
shock therapy. *See* electroconvulsive
    therapy
Skorodin, Bernard, 84
Slovinsky, Louis, 122–123
sodium amytal, 23
Sodium Pentothal, 19
Solomon, Kenneth, 42
Solomon, Meyer, 13
Spitzer, Robert, 34, 38–46, 54–55, 98, 102
SSRIs (selective serotonin reuptake
    inhibitors), 4, 130

STAR*D trial, 130
statistics, 15, 35, 38, 55, 81, 92, 108, 130
Stein, Harry, 123
stigma, 108
stimulants, 29
Stoudemire, Alan, 53, 71
Styron, William, 112, 122
substance abuse, 37, 88, 90, 99, 101, 104,
    122
suggestion, 21
suicide, 4, 8, 50, 53, 59, 69, 71–72, 75, 88,
    122
symptoms of depression, 3, 27–28, 32, 42,
    44–45

teenagers, 70, 110–111
Terman, Louis, 84
testosterone, 93
Thorazine. *See* chlorpromazine
Tomlinson, H. A., 77–78
tricyclic antidepressants, 34, 62, 66–67

unconscious conflict, 14, 60
Unfinished Business (Scarf), 116

vitamins, 62

war neuroses, 19–20
Washington University in St. Louis, 36, 40,
    98
Wayne, John, 112
Weissman, Myrna, 37, 52–53, 66, 91, 95,
    117
White, E. B., 58
White, William A., 82
Wiley, Harvey W., 120
Williams, Henry Smith, 17
Winokur, George, 40, 48, 95, 96
Woodruff, Robert, 35–36, 40, 131
World War II, 19–20, 22, 25

Young, Frank Fenwick, 84
Young, Robert, 122
youth crisis, 68–69

Ziszook, Sidney, 50
Zung depression scale, 101

About the Author

Laura Hirshbein completed her medical school and residency training at the University of Michigan, and completed her PhD in the history of medicine from the Johns Hopkins University Institute of the History of Medicine. She is currently a psychiatrist and historian at the University of Michigan.